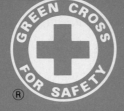

National Safety Council

First Aid and CPR

Second Edition

Level 2

The first aid and CPR procedures in this book are based on the most current recommendations of responsible medical sources. The National Safety Council and the publisher, however, make no guarantee as to, and assume no responsibility for, the correctness, sufficiency or completeness of such information or recommendations. Other or additional safety measures may be required under particular circumstances.

Library of Congress Cataloging-in-Publication Data

First aid and CPR : level 2 / National Safety council.—2nd ed.
        p.   cm.
    ISBN 0-86720-825-2
    1. First aid in illness and injury.   2. CPR (First aid)
I. National Safety Council.
RC86.7.F559   1993
616.02′52—dc20   93-21366
                                                            CIP

Eight records of fact reprinted with permission of the publisher, Guinness Publishing Ltd (copyright © 1989 Guinness Publishing Ltd), appear on pages 98, 118, 126, 127, and 178.

Vice President and Publisher ■ Clayton E. Jones
Assistant Editor ■ Heather Stratton
Production Editor ■ Anne Noonan
Design and Production ■ PC&F, Inc.
Cover Design ■ Hannus Design Associates

Principal Photographer ■ Rick Nye
Illustrations ■ Chris Young, artist
Greg Kyle, Larry Hall, Matt Hall, illustrators
Other full-color illustrations ■
  Bruce Argyle, M.D.
  H.B. Bectal, M.D.
  Michael D. Ellis
  Murray P. Hamlet, D.V.M.
  Axel W. Hoke, M.D.
  Sherman A. Minton, M.D.
  Eugene Robertson, M.D.
  Richard C. Ruffalo, D.M.D.
  Jeffrey Saffle, M.D.
  Clifford C. Snyder, M.D.
  Charles E. Stewart, M.D.
  Health Edco

Jones and Bartlett Publishers
40 Tall Pine Drive
Sudbury, MA 01776
(508) 443-5000
(800) 832-0034
info@jbpub.com
http://www.jbpub.com

Printed in the United States of America
97 96   10 9 8 7 6 5 4 3

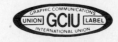

Welcome Message

Congratulations on your decision to take National Safety Council first aid training. More than 140,000 Americans die every year from injuries, and one in three suffers a nonfatal injury, so it is likely that at some time in your life you will encounter an emergency requiring first aid.

Your training in what to do and how to do it may help keep someone alive or prevent a more serious injury. Emergencies can happen anywhere and at any time.

We hope you will enjoy learning more about first aid through the careful study and application of the concepts being taught. Your training can make it possible for you to act confidently if someone needs help when seconds count.

It is wonderful to be able to save a life or aid someone who has been injured! Protecting life and promoting health have been the Council's only mission since 1913.

On behalf of the National Safety Council, as well as our local safety councils and training agencies, I wish you success in your first aid training program.

Sincerely,

Gerard F. Scannell, President
National Safety Council

Table of Contents

1

Introduction

Size of the Injury Problem

Injuries are one of the most serious public health problems. Injuries are the leading cause of death and disability in children and young adults. They destroy the health, lives, and livelihoods of millions of people.

- Each year, more than 140,000 Americans die from injuries (this includes accidents, suicides, and homicides), and one person in three suffers a nonfatal injury.
- Preceded by heart disease, cancer, and stroke, injury is the fourth leading cause of death among all Americans.
- One of every eight hospital beds is occupied by an injured patient.

Percentages of years of potential life lost to injury, cancer, heart disease, and other diseases before age 65. Modified from Centers for Disease Control.

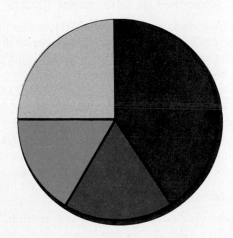

■ Heart Disease, 16.4%

■ Cancers, 18.0%

■ Injury, 40.8%

■ All other diseases, 24.8%

- Every year, more than 80,000 Americans suffer unnecessary but permanently disabling injuries of the brain or spinal cord.
- Injury is the leading reason for physician contacts. And more than 25% of hospital emergency room visits are for the treatment of injuries.

Need for First Aid Training

Because of the size and magnitude of the injury problem, everyone must expect sooner or later to be present when an injury or sudden illness strikes. The outcome of such misfortune frequently depends not only on the severity of the injury or illness, but on the first aid rendered. Therefore, every person should be trained in first aid.

First aid is the immediate care given to the injured or suddenly ill person. First aid does *not* take the place of proper medical treatment. It consists only of furnishing temporary assistance until competent medical care, *if needed,* is obtained, or until the chance for recovery without medical care is assured. *Most injuries and illnesses require only first aid care.*

Properly applied, first aid may mean the difference between life and death, rapid recovery and long hospitalization, or temporary disability and permanent injury.

Legal Aspects of First Aid

Duty to Act

No one is required to render aid when no legal duty to do so exists. For example, even a physician could ignore a stranger suffering a heart attack or a fractured bone. Moral obligations exist, but they may not be the same as a legal obligation to give aid.

Duty to act may occur in the following situations:

1. *When employment requires it.* If your employment has designated you to render first aid and you are called to an accident scene, then you have a duty to act. Examples include law enforcement officers, park rangers, lifeguards, and teachers who have a job description usually designating the giving of first aid.

2. *When a preexisting responsibility exists.* You may have a preexisting relationship with another person which demands being responsible for them (e.g., parent-child, driver-passenger) although it is not spelled out in your job description. You must give first aid should they need it.

3. *After beginning first aid.* Once you start first aid, you cannot stop. Duty to give first aid is usually questioned only when a person fails to act.

Standards of Care

Standards of care ensure quality care and protection for injured or suddenly sick victims. The elements making up a standard of care include:

1. *The type of rescuer.* A first aider should provide the level and type of care expected of a reasonable person with the same amount of training and in similar circumstances.

2. *Published recommendations.* Emergency care-related organizations and societies publish recommended first aid procedures. For example, the American Heart Association publishes procedures for giving CPR.

Obtain Consent to Help

You should obtain the victim's approval or permission before starting first aid. This permission is known as **consent.**

- When a victim gives permission to a first aider to help, this is known as **actual consent.** Oral or written permission is valid.
- Consent should be obtained from every conscious, mentally competent adult.
- Permission is implied for giving care for an unconscious victim and is known as **implied consent.** A first aider should not hesitate to treat an unconscious victim.
- Consent should be obtained from the parent or guardian of a victim who is a child, or of one who is an adult but is mentally incompetent. If a parent or guardian is not available, emergency first aid to maintain life may be given without consent. Do *not* withhold first aid from a minor just to obtain parental or guardian permission.
- Psychological emergencies present difficult problems of consent. Under most conditions, a police officer is the only person with the authority to restrain and transport a person against the person's will. However, if the victim is not violent, the situation is similar to that for minors.

Abandonment

Abandonment refers to the behavior of a first aider who begins giving care and then leaves the victim before another person arrives to take over. After starting first aid, you must remain with the victim until he or she is under the care of another person with equal or more training, or until the victim refuses treatment or transportation.

The Right to Refuse Care

A difficult problem involves the conscious, rational, adult victim who is suffering from an actual or potential life-threatening injury or illness but who refuses treatment or transportation. In such situations, make every reasonable effort to convince the victim, or anyone who can influence the victim, to accept first aid and/or transportation. When such a victim refuses to consent, do *not* give first aid or transportation. In such cases, document everything on paper, and if possible, have witnesses.

Parent Refusing Permission to Help a Child

Very rarely will a first aider encounter a parent who refuses permission—usually on moral, ethical, or religious grounds—to care for a seriously injured or ill child. If refusal does occur, make every effort to convince the parent about the seriousness of the problem and the necessity of first aid. If you do not succeed, call the police, document everything, and, if possible, have witnesses.

The Intoxicated or Belligerent Victim

If an intoxicated or belligerent victim refuses first aid, make every effort to persuade him or her of the need for such care. If refused, document everything in writing; if possible, have witnesses.

If the intoxicated person consents to first aid, take the greatest possible care. Alcohol and drugs may hide signs and symptoms of an injury. Because first aiders may be repulsed by the appearance and/or attitude of the intoxicated person, they may overlook injuries. It's important to focus on helping the victim.

Good Samaritan Laws

First aiders are covered by a Good Samaritan law in some states. Good Samaritan laws protect only those acting in good faith and without gross negligence or willful misconduct. If first aiders provide care within the scope of their training, lawsuits are rare. However, if a minor injury is worsened by a first aider, litigation is possible even if the first aider or medical person is covered by a Good Samaritan law. Actually, these laws provide no legal protection. Protection for a first aider consists of being properly trained and applying appropriate procedures and skills.

2

Victim Assessment

■ Primary Survey ■ Secondary Survey ■

Do *not* move the injured or suddenly ill person until you have a clear idea of the injury or illness and have applied first aid. The exception occurs when the victim is exposed to further danger at the accident scene. If the injury is serious, if it occurred in an area where the victim can remain safely, and if emergency medical service (EMS) attention is readily available, it is sometimes best not to attempt to move the person, but to use first aid at the injury scene until the EMS system responds.

When making a victim assessment, a first aider will consider what witnesses to the accident can tell about the accident, what is observed about the victim, and what the victim can tell.

The first aider must not assume that the obvious injuries are the only ones present because less noticeable injuries may also have occurred. Look for the causes of the injury which may provide a clue as to the extent of physical damage.

In all actions taken during the initial survey the first aider should be especially careful not to move the victim any more than necessary to support life. Any unnecessary movement or rough handling should be avoided because it might aggravate undetected fractures or spinal injuries.

In order to provide good first aid, a person should be able to identify a victim's injury or sudden illness and its seriousness. To find out what is wrong and how extensive it is, the first aider should follow a systematic approach known as a victim assessment.

A victim assessment attempts to:

■ Get the victim's consent
■ Gain the victim's confidence
■ Identify the victim's problem(s) and determine which of them requires immediate first aid
■ Get information about the victim that may prove useful later to the EMS responders and attending medical personnel

A victim assessment of either an injured victim or a medically ill victim is divided into two steps:

■ Primary survey
■ Secondary survey

Primary Survey

The primary survey covers these areas:

A—Airway open?
B—Breathing?
C—Circulation at carotid pulse?
H—Hemorrhage—severe bleeding?

The primary survey is the first step in assessing a victim. Its purpose is to find and correct life-threatening conditions.

Airway. Ask: Does the victim have an open airway? If the person is talking or is conscious, the airway is open. Refer to page 18 for the correct and detailed procedures for opening an airway.

Breathing. Ask: Is the victim breathing? Conscious victims are breathing. However, note any breathing difficulties or unusual breathing sounds. If the victim is unconscious, keep the airway open and *look* for the chest to rise and fall, *listen* for breathing, and *feel* for air coming out of the victim's nose and mouth. See page 18 for the correct and detailed procedures.

Circulation. Ask: Is the victim's heart beating? Determine this by feeling for a pulse at the side of the neck (carotid pulse). Refer to page 20 for the correct and detailed procedures.

Hemorrhage. Ask: Is the victim severely bleeding? Check for severe bleeding by looking, if necessary, over the victim's entire body for blood-soaked clothing as a sign of severe bleeding. See page 51 for the correct and detailed procedures.

Secondary Survey

Having completed the primary survey and attended to any life-threatening problems it uncovers, take a closer look at the victim and make a systematic assessment called the secondary survey.

Look for important signs and symptoms of injury. A **sign** is something the first aider sees, hears, or feels (e.g., pale face, no respiration, cool skin). A **symptom** is something the victim tells the first aider about (e.g.,

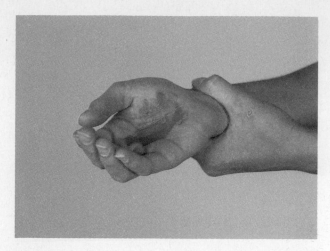

A sign

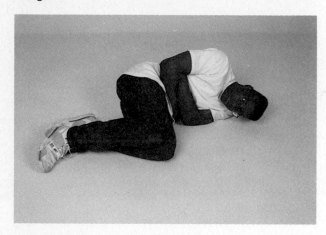

A symptom

nausea, back pain, no sensation in the extremities).

The secondary survey is done to discover problems that do not pose an immediate threat to life but may do so if they remain uncorrected. The secondary survey has three parts:

- Interview
- Vital signs
- Head-to-Toe Exam

Interview

First, identify yourself and get the victim's consent for you to give first aid. See page 2 for more information on consent and its legal implications.

The interview usually involves only the victim. Start by introducing yourself and asking for the victim's name (use it during the assessment). Get the victim's consent before giving first aid. In some cases the victim's family and any bystanders may be involved. Ask the victim about his or her chief complaint. Often it is obvious (e.g., bleeding). Most chief complaints are characterized by pain or an abnormal function.

For an unconscious victim, monitor breathing and pulse, and if needed, render rescue breathing or CPR.

After finding out about the chief complaint and if

time permits, two mnemonic devices might help you identify a victim's problem: taking a S-A-M-P-L-E history and, since pain is one of the most common chief complaints, using P-A-I-N as a way of describing the victim's pain:

> **S**ymptoms (chief complaint)
> **A**llergies (may give a clue as to the problem)
> **M**edications (may give a clue as to the problem)
> **P**reexisting illnesses (relating to the problem)
> **L**ast food (in case of needed surgery, or case of food poisoning)
> **E**vents prior to the injury
>
> **P**eriod of pain (How long? What started it?)
> **A**rea (Where?)
> **I**ntensity (How strong?)
> **N**ullify (What stops it? such as rest, certain position)

Vital Signs

First aiders involve themselves with the following vital signs: pulse, respirations, and, if indicated, skin condition. Check these every five or so minutes while waiting for the EMS to respond or while transporting the victim to a medical facility.

Pulse. Place two fingertips (do *not* use a thumb since it has its own pulse) over either the radial pulse point (on thumb side of inside wrist) or the carotid pulse point (in the groove beside the Adam's apple on the neck). Do *not* feel both carotid arteries at the same time. Do *not* put too much pressure on or massage the carotid artery area because either will disturb the heart's rhythm.

Normal pulse at rest for adults is from 60 to 80 beats per minute. For children, it is 80 to 100; and for babies, it is 100 to 140 beats per minute.

TABLE 2–1 Normal Pulse Rates	
60–70	Men
70–80	Women
80–90	Children over seven years
80–120	Children from one to seven years
110–130	Infants
Pulse Classified in Adults	
60 and below	Slow or subnormal
60–80	Normal (men, women)
80–100	Moderate increase
100–120	Quick
120–140	Rapid
140 and above	Running (hard to count)

Source: U.S. Public Health Service, The Ship's Medicine Chest and Medical Aid at Sea.

TABLE 2-2 What Body Temperatures Mean

Fahrenheit (F)		Centigrade (C)
108°	Usually fatal	42.2°
107 ⌉		⌐ 41.7
106 ⎬	Critical condition	⎬ 41.1
105 ⌋		⌊ 40.6
104 ⌉		⌐ 40.0
103 ⎬	High fever	⎬ 39.4
102 ⌋		⌊ 38.9
101 ⌉		⌐ 38.3
100 ⎬	Moderate fever	⎬ 37.8
99 ⌋		⌊ 37.2
98.6	Healthy (normal) temperature in mouth	37.0
98 ⌉		⌐ 36.7
97 ⎬	Subnormal	⎬ 36.1
96 ⎬	temperature	⎬ 35.6
95 ⌋		⌊ 35.0

Source: U.S. Public Health Service. The Ship's Medicine Chest and Medical Aid at Sea.

Respiration. During the primary survey, the concern focused upon "Is the victim breathing?" However, in the secondary survey, the respiration rate is determined.

Count the number of breaths per minute. Between 12 and 20 breaths per minute is normal for resting adults and older children. Up to 30 breaths per minute is normal for children, and 40 is normal for babies.

As you determine the respiration rate, listen for sounds, for example:

- A whistle or wheeze—constricted airway
- A crowing sound—constricted airway
- A gurgling sound—fluid in airway
- A snoring sound—tongue blockage

Skin Condition. Skin condition refers to two things:

- **Temperature.** Body temperature is best taken with a thermometer. Often one is not available. If such is the case, get an idea of the temperature by putting the back of one hand on the victim's forehead and the other on your own or that of another healthy person. If the victim has a fever, you should feel the difference. Fingertips and palms may be insensitive because of calluses.
- **Color.** Skin color, especially in light-skinned people, reflects the circulation under the skin as well as oxygen status. In darkly pigmented people, these changes may not be apparent in the skin, but may be assessed by examining the mucous membranes (inside mouth, inner eyelids, and nailbeds). If the skin's blood vessels constrict or pulse slows, the skin becomes pale, mottled, or cyanotic (bluish discoloration). If the skin's blood vessels dilate or blood flow increases, the skin becomes warm and pink.

Head-to-Toe Exam

The victim assessment's final step involves a head-to-toe exam. It consists of looking for other injuries. Tell the victim what is being done and why. Do *not* aggravate injuries or contaminate wounds. Do *not* move the victim in case of neck and spinal injuries. Removing of clothing from the victim during this exam is *not* usually necessary.

Head and Neck. Check the scalp for bleeding or deformity ("goose egg" or depression). Do *not* move the head during this procedure. Check the ears and nose for a clear fluid or bloody discharge. Look in the mouth for blood or foreign materials.

Eyes. Pay attention to pupil size—constricted or dilated. Look for unequal pupils. Use a flashlight to determine if the pupils are reactive. If there is no flashlight, cover the eye with your hand and notice the pupil reaction when the eye is uncovered. No pupil reaction to light could mean death, coma, cataracts in older persons, or an artificial eye. Look at the inner eyelid surface—pink is normal in all healthy people regardless of skin pigmentation. A pale color may indicate anemia or blood loss.

Chest. Check the chest for cuts, bruises, penetrations, and impaled objects. Warn the victim that you are going to apply pressure to the sides of the chest. Pain from squeezing or compressing the sides may indicate a rib fracture.

Abdomen. Anything protruding from the abdomen will be obvious, but check for penetrating objects. If a chief complaint is abdominal pain, ask the victim to point to where it hurts. Then, beginning on the opposite side from the spot, press gently on different parts

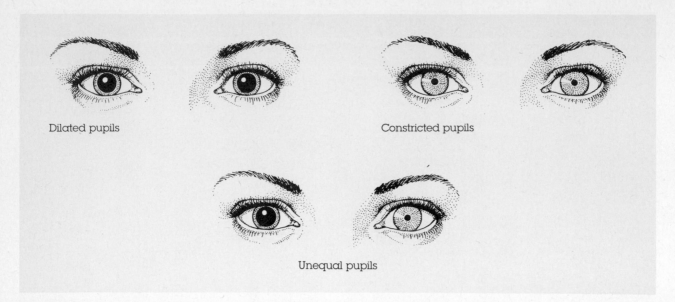

Dilated pupils

Constricted pupils

Unequal pupils

Changes in pupil size can have medical significance.

of the abdomen to see where it hurts the most. Feel for abnormal lumps and hardened areas. Do *not* push too deeply. The victim may "guard" an area if it is tender by tightening abdominal muscles or protecting that area with his or her hands. Feel the four abdominal quadrants. (Divide the abdomen into four parts by two imaginary lines intersecting at right angles at the navel.)

Extremity Assessment. Check the arms and legs for injury, deformity and tenderness. Compare the two sides of the body with each other. Blood circulation can be checked by feeling the pulse, the warmth of the part, and capillary refill in a nailbed. To assess capillary refill, gently press on the nailbed's surface to whiten the underlying tissue. Then, release the pressure and observe the rate at which the nailbed becomes pink again. Instant refilling indicates good circulation. Refill time greater than two seconds is definitely abnormal. Check the radial pulse (in the wrist) and the pedal pulse (on the ankle or the top of the foot) for blood circulation.

Spine and Back Assessment. Help the victim avoid excessive movement. In a victim with possible spinal injury as well as one with suspected stroke, check sensation and strength in all extremities by pressing his or her foot against your hand. The spinal injured victim may show paraplegia (paralysis of both legs) or quadriplegia (paralysis of all four extremities); the stroke victim is likely to have hemiplegia (paralysis of an arm or leg on the same side of the body).

Putting It All Together

The victim assessment will be influenced by whether the victim is suffering from a medical problem or an injury, whether the victim is conscious or unconscious, and whether life-threatening conditions are present. Remember to first conduct a primary survey and correct any problems it uncovers before going on to the secondary survey.

Medical Alert Tag

A medical alert emblem tag worn as a necklace or as a bracelet attracts attention in an emergency situation. These tags contain the wearer's medical problem and a 24-hour telephone number to call in case of an emergency. Do *not* remove a medical alert tag from an injured or sick person.

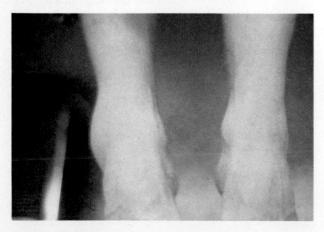

Sprained ankle

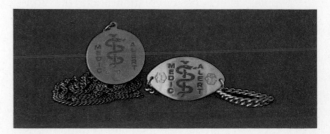

Medical alert tag

TABLE 2-3 Diagnostic Signs

Observation	Examples
Pulse	
Rapid, strong	fright, apprehension, heat stroke
Rapid, weak	shock, bleeding, diabetic coma, heat exhaustion
Slow, strong	stroke, skull fracture
None	cardiac arrest, death
Respirations	
Shallow	shock, bleeding, heat exhaustion, insulin shock
Deep, gasping, labored	airway obstruction, chest injury, diabetic coma, heart disease
None	respiratory arrest due to any number of illnesses/injuries
Bright, frothy blood coughed up	lung damage possible due to fractured ribs or penetrating objects
Skin temperature	
Cool, moist	shock, bleeding, heat exhaustion
Cool, dry	exposure to cold
Hot, dry	heat stroke, high fever
Face color	
Red	high blood pressure, heat stroke, diabetic coma
Pale/white/ashen	shock, bleeding, heat exhaustion, insulin shock
Blue	heart failure, airway obstruction, some poisonings

Note: Blue results from poor oxygenation of circulating blood. For people with dark skin pigmentation, blue may be noted around the fingernails, palms of hands and mouth.

Observation	Examples
Pupils of eyes	
Dilated	shock, bleeding, heat stroke, cardiac arrest
Constricted	opiate addiction
Unequal	head injury, stroke
State of consciousness	
Confusion	most any illness/injury, fright, apprehension, alcohol, drugs
Coma	stroke, head injury, severe poisoning, diabetic coma
Inability to move upon command (an indicator of paralysis)	
One side of the body	stroke, head injury
Arms and legs	damage to spinal cord in neck
Legs	damage to spinal cord below neck
Reaction to physical stimulation (an indicator of paralysis)	
No sensation in arms and/or legs	damage to spinal cord as indicated above
Numbness in arms and/or legs	damage to spinal cord as indicated above

Note: No sensation or indication of pain when there is an obvious injury can also be due to hysteria, violent shock, or excessive alcohol or drug use.

Source: National Highway Traffic Safety Administration, Emergency Medical Services: First Responder Training Course (Washington, D.C.: U.S. Superintendent of Documents).

Calling the Emergency Medical Services (EMS) System for Help*

In many communities, to receive emergency assistance of every kind you just dial 9-1-1. Check to see if this is true in your community. An emergency number should be listed on the inside cover of your telephone directory.

To receive the best emergency medical help fast, you should keep a list of phone numbers for important services near your telephone.

1. ***The rescue squad.*** Often part of the local fire department, these specially trained paramedics are likely to respond swiftly and competently.

2. ***The police.*** They may or may not be able to

Adapted from Consumer's Union, Consumer's Reports.

TABLE 2–4 Victim Assessment

Scene Survey

- dangerous hazards?   - number of victims?   - cause of injury?

Primary Survey (also known as Basic Life Support (BLS))

Check responsiveness/protect spine

A = Airway open? (head-tilt/chin-lift)
B = Breathing? (look at chest; listen and feel for air)
C = Circulation? (pulse at carotid?)
H = Hemorrhage? (severe bleeding; personal protection)

Secondary Survey

Interview

- Introduce self/reassure/victim's name/obtain consent/ask questions:

    S = Signs/Symptoms (chief complaint)?
        P = Period of pain (how long)?
        A = Area (where)?
        I = Intensity?
        N = Nullify (what stops it)?
    A = Allergies?
    M = Medications currently taking?
    P = Pertinent past medical history?
    L = Last oral intake: solid or liquid? when and how much?
    E = Events leading to injury or illness?

Vital signs

- Pulse: rate?
- Respiration: rate/sounds?
- Skin condition: temperature/color/moisture?
- Capillary refill?

Head-to-Toe Examination (use **LAF**: L = Look; A = Ask; F = Feel)

Head:	- Bleeding/deformity/CSF (ears/nose)/mouth clear/cyanosis?
Eyes:	- Pupils: equal & react to light (PEARL)/inner eyelid color?
Chest:	- Wounds/penetrating object?
	- Pain (with/without rib spring)?
Abdomen:	- Wounds/penetrating object?
	- Pain/guarding/rigidity (with/without gentle pushing)?
Extremities:	- Wounds/deformity/tenderness (compare 2 sides)?
	- pulses?
	- capillary refill?
Spinal cord:	- Finger/toe wiggle?
	- Touch finger/toe for sensation?
	- Hand squeeze/foot push?

Medical Alert Tag?

respond with medically trained personnel; however, they can get someone to the hospital quickly.

3. _Ambulance service._ Some services have trained paramedics; others do not.

4. _Your doctor._ Your own doctor may not be available, but he or she should be alerted if an emergency has occurred.

5. _Poison control center._ In some communities, this service will give information to doctors only. Call before an emergency occurs to find out.

Give the following information over the phone:

1. _The victim's location._ Give city or town, street name, and street number. Give names of intersecting streets or roads and other landmarks if possible. Describe the building. The victim's location may be the single most important information you can provide.

2. _Your phone number._ This information is required not only to help prevent false calls but, more importantly, to allow the center to call back for additional information.

3. _What has happened._ Tell the nature of the emergency (traffic accident, heart attack, dog bite, and so on).

4. _Number of persons needing help and any special conditions._ Tell the number of people involved. Tell about any special problems, such as several flights of stairs and no elevators, or the presence of a guard dog.

5. _Condition of the victim(s)._ Tell about such things as no breathing or pulse, severe bleeding, unconsciousness.

6. _What is being done for the victim(s)._ Tell about CPR, how the bleeding is being controlled, and so on.

Always be the last to hang up the phone. The EMS system dispatcher may need to ask more questions about how to find you. They may also tell you what to do until help arrives.

Speak slowly and clearly. Shouting is difficult to understand.

According to the National Emergency Number Association, 75% of the population and 25% of the geographic area in the United States have 9–1–1 coverage. Record your local community emergency telephone numbers and other information on this book's back cover.

Triage

You may encounter emergency situations with two or more victims. This is often the case in multiple car ac-

cidents or disasters. After making a quick scene survey, it is necessary to decide who is to be cared for and transported first. This process of prioritizing or classifying injured victims is called "triage." Triage is a French word meaning "to sort." The goal is to do the greatest good for the greatest number of victims.

Finding Life-Threatened Victims

A variety of systems are used to identify care and transportation priorities. To find those needing immediate care for life-threatening conditions, follow these steps:

Step #1: Tell all people who can get up and walk to move to a specific area. If victims can get up and walk, they rarely have life-threatening injuries. These victims ("the walking wounded") are classified as delayed priority (see below). Do not force the victim to move if he or she complains of pain.

Step #2: Find the life-threatened victims by performing only the primary survey on all remaining victims. Go to the motionless victims first. You must move rapidly (less than 60 seconds per victim) from one victim to the next until all have been assessed. Classify victims according to these care and transportation priorities:

1. _Immediate care:_ Victim has life-threatening injuries but can be saved.
- Airway or breathing difficulties (not breathing or breathing rate faster than 30 per minute)
- Weak or no pulse
- Uncontrolled or severe bleeding
- Unresponsive or unconscious

2. _Urgent care:_ Victims not fitting into the immediate or delayed categories. Care and transportation can be delayed up to one hour.

3. _Delayed care:_ victims with minor injuries. Care and transportation can be delayed up to three hours.

4. _Dead:_ victims are obviously dead, mortally wounded, or unlikely to survive because of the extent of their injuries, age, and medical condition.

Do not become involved in treating the victims at this point, but ask knowledgeable bystanders to care for immediate life-threatening problems (i.e., rescue breathing, bleeding control).

Step #3: Reassess victims regularly for changes in their condition. Only after the immediate life-threatening conditions receive care should those with less serious conditions be given care.

Later, you will usually be relieved when more highly trained emergency personnel arrive on the scene. You may be asked to provide first aid, to help move, or to help with ambulance or helicopter transportation.

■ PRIMARY SURVEY ■

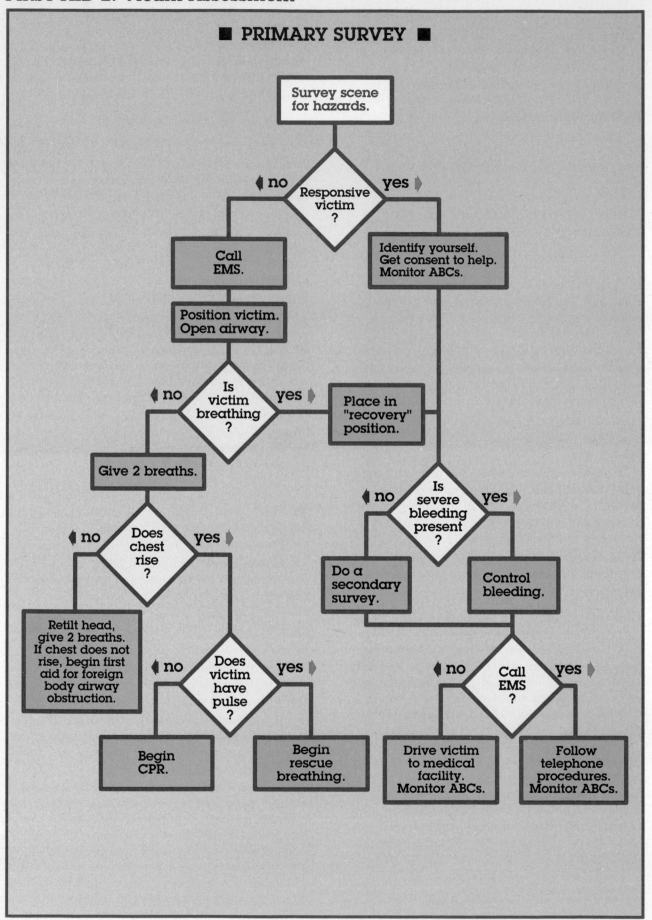

Survey scene for hazards.

Responsive victim?
- no
- yes

no →

Call EMS.

Position victim. Open airway.

Is victim breathing?
- no
- yes

Give 2 breaths.

Does chest rise?
- no
- yes

Retilt head, give 2 breaths. If chest does not rise, begin first aid for foreign body airway obstruction.

Does victim have pulse?
- no
- yes

Begin CPR.

Begin rescue breathing.

yes →

Identify yourself. Get consent to help. Monitor ABCs.

Place in "recovery" position.

Is severe bleeding present?
- no
- yes

Do a secondary survey.

Control bleeding.

Call EMS?
- no
- yes

Drive victim to medical facility. Monitor ABCs.

Follow telephone procedures. Monitor ABCs.

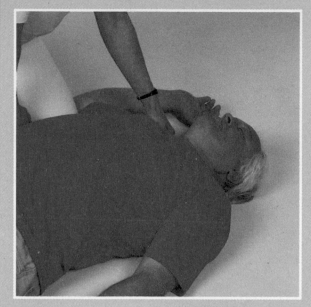

Responsive?

A = Airway open?

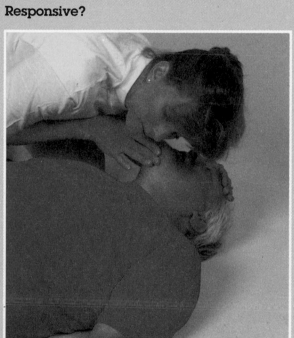

B = Breathing?

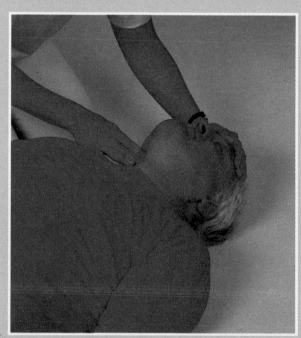

C = Circulation at carotid pulse?

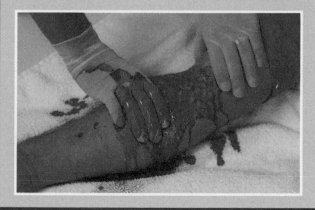

H = Hemorrhage—severe bleeding?

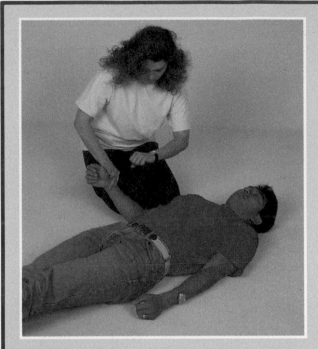

Pulse rate: Radial

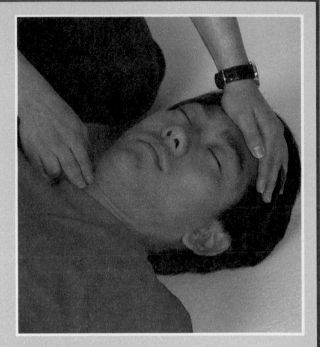

Pulse rate: Carotid

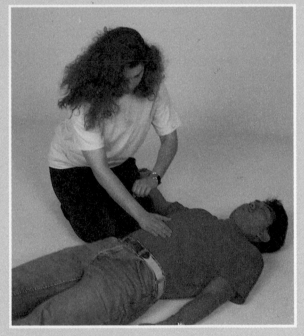

Respiration rate

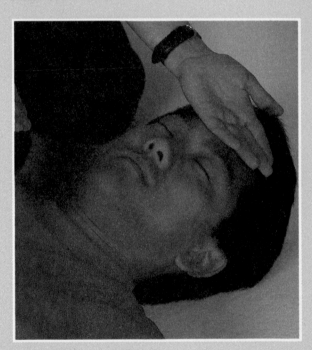

Skin temperature

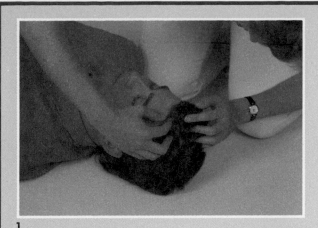

1.

1. Check scalp and head for bleeding or deformity. Do not move head.

2. Check ears and nose for clear fluid or blood.

3. Check mouth for blood or foreign materials.

4. Check pupils for size, equality, and reaction.

5. Check inner eyelid color.

6. Check chest for wounds.

7. Squeeze sides of chest for tenderness.

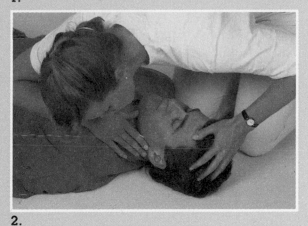

2.

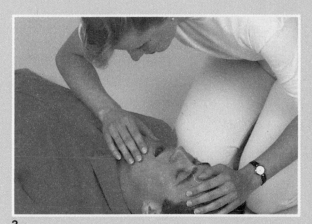

3.

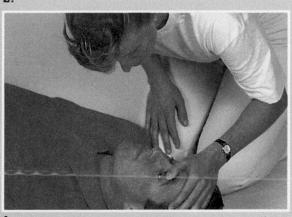

4.

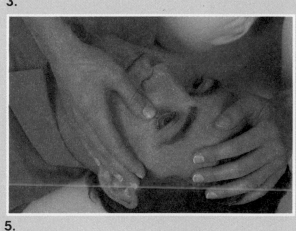

5.

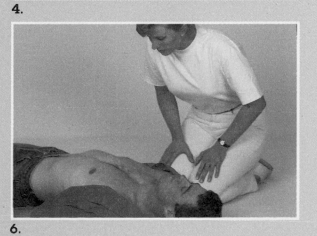

6.

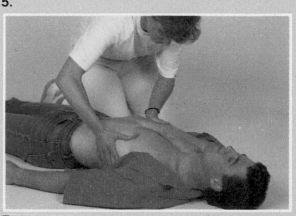

7.

SKILL SCAN: Head-to-Toe Exam

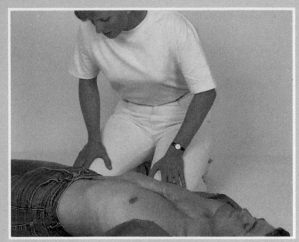

8.

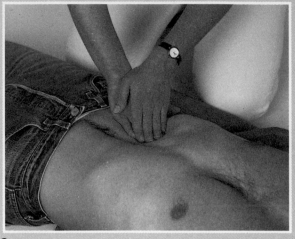

9.

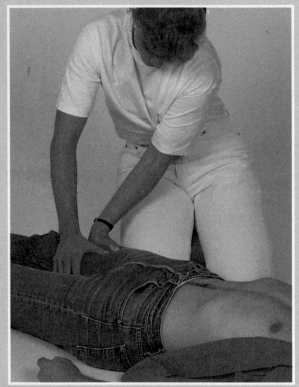

10.

8. Check abdomen for wounds.

9. Gently press abdomen for tenderness.

10. Check arms and legs for deformity and tenderness. Compare two sides with each other.

11. Pinch fingernail or toenail (capillary refill test).

12A and B. Check pulses.

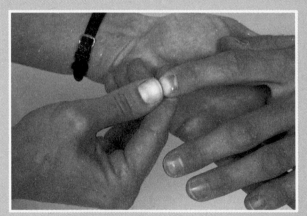

11.

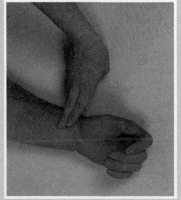

12A.

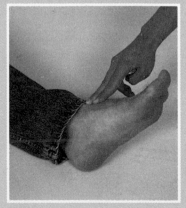

12B.

■ ACTIVITY 1 ■
Victim Assessment

Mark each statement true (T) or false (F).

1. _____ If you find severe bleeding during a victim evaluation, continue your examination and come back to the bleeding later.

2. _____ Use your thumb to feel for a victim's pulse.

3. _____ A pulse can be felt at either the wrist's radial point or the neck's carotid point.

4. _____ Feel for both carotid points at the same time.

5. _____ Normal adult pulse rate is 60–80 beats per minute.

6. _____ Normal adult respiration rate is between 12 and 20 breaths per minute.

7. _____ Clear fluid draining from the nose or ears may be cerebrospinal fluid (CSF).

8. _____ Very small (pinpointed) eye pupils can mean a state of shock.

9. _____ Unequal eye pupils may result from a head injury.

10. _____ All normal, healthy people (regardless of skin color) have a pink inner eyelid surface.

11. _____ The capillary refill technique can indicate the quality of blood circulation in an arm or leg.

Designate the following as signs (A) or symptoms (B).

1. _____ Sherry states that she feels dizzy.

2. _____ Matt says he feels like throwing up.

3. _____ Steve's skin is red and blistered.

4. _____ Jim says that he has no feeling in his right arm.

5. _____ Scott's pulse rate is 88 beats per minute.

6. _____ Joni's oral temperature is 104°F.

7. _____ Justin's pupils are unequal.

8. _____ Mike begins to vomit.

9. _____ Blood is spurting from Tom's leg.

10. _____ Carla has a fruity odor on her breath.

11. _____ Glen has an impaled object in his eye.

12. _____ Cerebrospinal fluid is coming from Joann's ear.

13. _____ Wes has a deformity in his wrist after falling on it.

14. _____ Liz is wheezing while breathing.

15. _____ After falling, Whitney's ankle becomes swollen.

3

Basic Life Support*

■ What is CPR? ■ Foreign Body Airway Obstruction ■ Disease Precautions ■
■ CPR Performance Mistakes ■ Remembering the Steps of CPR ■

What Is CPR?

Cardiopulmonary resuscitation (CPR) combines rescue breathing (also known as mouth-to-mouth breathing) and external chest compressions. *Cardio* refers to the heart and *pulmonary* refers to the lungs. *Resuscitation* refers to revive. Proper and prompt CPR serves as a holding action by providing oxygen to the brain and heart until advanced cardiac life support (ACLS) can be provided.

Need for CPR Training

Heart disease causes more than half the deaths in North America. About two-thirds of these deaths are from heart attacks, and more than half of these were dead on arrival (DOA) at a hospital. Sudden death related to heart attacks is the most prominent medical emergency in the United States today.

It is possible that a large number of these deaths could be prevented by prompt action to provide rapid entry into the EMS system, prompt CPR, and early defibrillation. CPR can save heart attack victims, and it can also save lives in cases of drowning, suffocation, electrocution, and drug overdose. Use CPR any time a victim's breathing and heart have stopped. Use rescue breathing whenever there is a pulse but no breathing.

When to Start CPR

Trained people need to be able to:

■ Recognize the signs of cardiac arrest
■ Provide CPR, and
■ Call for the emergency medical services (EMS).

Most people suffering a fatal heart attack die within two hours of the first signs and symptoms of the attack.

Activate the EMS system and start CPR as soon as possible! Victims have a good chance of surviving if:

■ CPR is started within the first four minutes of heart stoppage, and
■ They receive advanced cardiac life support within the next four minutes.

Brain damage begins after four to six minutes and is certain after ten minutes when no CPR is given.

Activating the EMS System

Call the local emergency telephone number, usually 9-1-1. The caller should be ready to give the EMS dispatcher the following information:

■ *The victim's location.* Give address, names of intersecting streets or roads and other landmarks if possible.
■ *Your phone number.* This prevents false calls, and allows the center to call back for additional information if needed.
■ *What happened.* Tell the nature of the emergency (e.g., heart attack, drowning, etc.)
■ *Number of persons needing help and any special conditions.*

*Based on the 1992 American Heart Association, Guidelines for Cardiopulmonary Resuscitation and Emergency Cardiac Care, JAMA, 1992; 268:2172

TABLE 3-1 Chances of Survival (Survival Rate %)

		Time Until Advanced Cardiac Life Support Begins		
		<8 min.	8–16 min.	>16 min.
Time Until Basic Life Support (CPR)	<4 min.	43%	19%	10%
	4–8 min.	27%	19%	6%
	>8 min.	N/A	7%	0%

Source: National Ski Patrol, based upon Eisenberg, et. al., JAMA, 1979; 241:1905–1907.

- **The victim's condition** (e.g., conscious, breathing, etc.) **and what is being done for the victim** (tell about CPR, rescue breathing). **Always be the last to hang up the phone!**

Moving a Victim

Do **not** move a victim even in cramped, busy locations until effective CPR is given and qualified help arrives. If endangered by hazards, such as a potential landslide, cave-in, or burning building, move to safe area before starting CPR.

Signs of Successful CPR

Successful CPR refers to correct CPR performance, not victim survival. Even with successful CPR, most victims will not survive unless they receive advanced cardiac life support (e.g., defibrillation, oxygen, and drug therapy). CPR serves as a holding action until such medical care can be provided. Early bystander CPR (started in less than four minutes after cardiac arrest) coupled with an EMS system with advanced cardiac life support capability (within eight minutes) can increase survival chances to more than 40 percent.

Check CPR's effectiveness by:

- Watching chest rise and fall with each rescue breath
- Checking pulse after first minute of CPR and every few minutes afterward to determine if a pulse has returned.
- Having a second rescuer feel for carotid pulse while giving chest compressions. A pulse should be felt each time a compression is made. If alone, do not try to give compressions with one hand while checking for a pulse at the same time.

When to Stop CPR

Stop resuscitation efforts when any of the following occurs:

- Victim revives (regains pulse and breathing). Though hoped for, most victims also require advanced cardiac procedures before they regain their heart and lung functions.
- Replaced by either another trained rescuer or EMS system
- Too exhausted to continue
- Scene becomes unsafe
- A physician tells you to stop.
- Cardiac arrest lasts longer than 30 minutes (with or without CPR). This suggestion is controversial, but is supported by the National Association of Emergency Medical Services Physicians.

Recovery Position

For an unconscious, breathing, uninjured victim, use the "recovery position":

- Roll victim onto side (if no evidence of head or neck injury)
- Place hand of upper arm under chin to support it
- Flex leg to prevent rolling

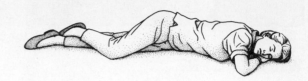

What about the Victim's Clothing?

Usually it's not necessary to remove or loosen victim's clothing. Remove or loosen clothing if:

- Collar does not allow feeling carotid pulse;
- Heavy clothing does not allow locating the notch at the sternum's tip
- Unable to find correct hand position
- Your locale allows EMS personnel to remove by cutting, ripping, or pulling up a victim's clothing in order to bare the chest. This includes either cutting a woman's bra or slipping it up to her neck.

How Does CPR Work?

Chest compressions and/or direct heart compression create enough pressure within the chest cavity to cause blood to move through the heart and circulatory system. Effective chest compressions provide only one-fourth to one-third of normal blood flow. Rescue breaths provide 16 percent oxygen content—enough to sustain life.

Why CPR May Fail to Resuscitate

During the early days of CPR (the 1970s), it was commonly believed that it would save a lot of lives. As it has turned out, it does not unless advanced cardiac life support quickly follows.

Only 15 percent of people who receive CPR live to go home from the hospital. Some of the reasons for CPR's failure:

- Delay in starting CPR
- Using improper techniques
- Victim had terminal or unmanageable disease (such as a massive heart attack)
- Delay in the victim receiving defibrillation—an electric jolt to the heart. CPR is a holding action until defibrillation which jump-starts the heart can be given to the victim.

When *NOT* to Start CPR

Usually start CPR whenever pulselessness occurs. However, do not start CPR if positive signs of death appear:

- Severe mutilation
- Rigor mortis
- Evidence of tissue decomposition
- Lividity (purple-reddish color showing on parts of body closest to ground)

Do not start CPR if evidence exists that the victim has been in cardiac arrest for more than 30 minutes withour prior resuscitation efforts. Exceptions include cold water drowning victims.

Do not start CPR when "do not resuscitate" orders apply—usually in writing and decided upon by victim's family and physician.

Do not start CPR in an unsafe environment or situation. In such cases and if possible, move the victim to a safe location and then begin CPR.

How Can an Untrained Rescuer Help

An untrained rescuer can help by:

- Going for help
- Checking breathing and pulse following directions from trained rescuer
- Performing CPR following directions from trained rescuer

If trained rescuer is exhausted, an untrained rescuer can give chest compressions while the trained rescuer gives rescue breaths. The trained rescuer can explain what to do. Instructions would include:

- Finding the proper hand position
- Keeping the fingers off victim's chest
- Keeping the arms straight and shoulders over victim's chest
- Performing five chest compressions at proper rate and depth, stopping while trained rescuer gives one breath, then having the untrained rescuer start another cycle with five chest compressions.

If the untrained rescuer adequately performs chest compressions, allow him/her to continue helping you.

Excuses Given by Some People for *NOT* Giving CPR

Sometimes a person may not want to provide help to a victim in distress. As discussed in Chapter 1, if a person has a duty to act (e.g., police, firefighter, lifeguard, teacher, etc.), they are required by law to render aid. But a layperson with no prior relationship to the victim or employment obligation may choose to ignore a victim's distress. Some people justify not helping a cardiac arrest victim by using various excuses. Their excuses may include one or more of the following:

- Claim they are unable to remember exact techniques
- Believe their training is old and without the latest methods their efforts would be ineffective.
- Afraid of injuring victim (e.g., breaking ribs)
- Fear a lawsuit (no one who has given CPR has been successfully sued)
- Believe only medical personnel should give CPR
- Fear of becoming infected by HIV which results in AIDS, hepatitis B (HBV), or other infectious disease
- Repulsed by the situation—presence of vomit, blood, odors, protective dogs, dangerous conditions
- Have a negative image of victim (examples: poorly dressed, poor personal hygiene, drunkenness)

Dangerous Complications of CPR

Vomiting may occur during CPR. If it happens it is usually before CPR has begun or within the first minute after beginning CPR. Inhaling vomit (aspiration) into the lungs can produce a type of pneumonia that can kill even after successful rescue efforts.

In case of vomiting:

1. Turn victim onto his/her side and keep there until vomiting ends.

2. Wipe vomit out of victim's mouth with your fingers wrapped in a cloth.

3. Reposition victim onto his/her back and resume rescue breathing/CPR if needed.

Stomach (gastric) distention describes stomach bulging from air. It is especially common in children.

- Caused by:
    1. Rescue breaths given too fast
    2. Rescue breaths given too forcefully
    3. Partially or completely blocked airway
- Dangerous because:
    1. Air in stomach pushes against lungs, making it difficult or impossible to give full breaths
    2. Possibility of inhaling vomit into the lungs
- Prevent or minimize by:
    1. Trying to blow just hard enough to make chest rise
    2. Keeping the airway open during inhalations and exhalations
    3. Using mouth-to-nose method

4. Slow rescue breathing—one-and-a-half to two seconds each—pause between breaths so you can take another breath

5. Retilting head to open airway

Inhalation of foreign substances (known as aspiration). Foreign substances have no place in the lungs. Three types of substances can create potentially life-threatening situations:

- Particulate matter aspiration—can stop-up airway
- Nongastric liquid aspiration—mainly due to fresh- and salt-water drowning
- Gastric acid aspiration—effects of gastric acid on lung tissue can be equated with a chemical burn.

Help prevent vomiting by placing victim on his/her left side. This position keeps the stomach from spilling its contents into esophagus by keeping the bottom end of esophagus (located where it enters the stomach) above the stomach.

Chest compression-related injuries can happen even with proper compressions. Injuries may include: rib fractures, rib separation, air and/or blood in chest cavity, bruised lung, lacerations of the lung, liver, or spleen.

Prevent or minimize by:

- Using proper hand location on chest—if too low the sternum's tip can cut into liver
- Keeping fingers off victim's ribs by interlocking fingers
- Pressing straight down instead of sideways
- Giving smooth, regular, and uninterrupted (except when breathing) compressions. Avoid sudden, jerking, jabbing, or stabbing compressions.
- Avoiding pressing chest too deeply

Dentures, loose or broken teeth, or dental appliances. Leave tight-fitting dentures in place to support victim's mouth during rescue breathing. Remove loose or broken teeth, dentures, and/or dental appliances.

Wilderness CPR

Since a cardiac arrest victim's heart activity must be restored within a short time (requires defibrillation and medications) for survival, CPR has limited use in the wilderness or a remote setting. This is especially true if severe trauma (i.e., massive head or chest injury, severe blood loss, severed spinal cord) accompanies cardiac arrest. Also, CPR is very difficult to continue during a wilderness evacuation.

Rescue breathing can be continued for hours when there is a pulse, but chest compressions cannot support circulation for a long time period. The National Association of Emergency Medical Services Physicians gives these guidelines for victims with normal core body temperatures or mild hypothermia (core body temperature above 90°F):

- If the victim is not breathing, give rescue breathing; if no pulse can be felt, give CPR.
- If the victim has been in cardiac arrest for more than 30 minutes without prior resuscitation efforts, do not start CPR.
- If CPR is given unsuccessfully for more than 30 minutes, stop CPR (see exceptions below).

The National Association of Emergency Medical Services Physicians recommends starting and continuing CPR for more than 30 minutes in the following situations:

- Cold water immersion of less than one hour. Hypothermia and possibly the mammalian diving reflex slows metabolism.
- Avalanche burial
- Hypothermia
- Lightning struck

Hypothermia

For the severe or profound hypothermic victim, CPR should not delay evacuation to a location for rewarming and advanced cardiac life support. Rough handling or CPR chest compressions can cause a form of heart attack (ventricular fibrillation). Therefore, be sure that there is no pulse before starting CPR. The American Heart Association guidelines suggest taking 30 to 45 seconds to feel for a pulse in an unresponsive hypothermic victim. Whereas, the National Association of Emergency Medical Services Physicians recommends taking at least one to two minutes to feel for the presence of a carotid pulse in the unresponsive hypothermic victim. Determining the existence of a pulse is difficult in cold environments because: (1) of the victim's very slow pulse rate and (2) the cold environment makes the pulse difficult to feel because of the rescuer's cold fingers.

The National Association of Emergency Medical Services Physicians' guidelines for a severe or profound hypothermic victim (core body temperature below 90°F are:

- Do *not* start CPR if:

  1. Core temperature is less than 60°F.

  2. Chest is frozen and cannot be compressed.

  3. Victim has been submersed for more than one hour.

  4. Obvious lethal injury is present.

  5. Procedures significantly delay evacuation to controlled rewarming location.

  6. The procedures put rescuers at risk.

- Stop CPR if:

  1. Rescuers are exhausted.

2. Procedures place rescuers at risk.

3. Procedures cause significant delays in evacuation to controlled rewarming location.

Foreign Body Airway Obstruction (Choking)

The National Safety Council reports more than 3,000 choking deaths yearly.

Types of Upper Airway Obstructions

Tongue: Unconsciousness produces relaxation of soft tissues. The tongue can fall into the airway. The idea that one has "swallowed his or her tongue" is impossible, but is explained by the slippage of the relaxed tongue into the airway. The tongue is the most common airway obstruction.

Vomit: Most people vomit when at or near death. Additional discussion about vomit appears elsewhere in this book.

Foreign Body: People, especially children, have inhaled all kinds of objects. Nuts, candy, hot dogs, and grapes are major offenders because of their shape and consistencies. Unconscious victim's airways can also be obstructed by a foreign body (i.e., vomit, teeth). Methods of removing a foreign object appear later in this chapter.

Swelling: Allergic reactions (anaphylaxis) and irritants (i.e., smoke, chemicals) can cause swelling. Even a nonallergic person who gets stung inside the throat by a bee, yellow jacket, or other flying insect can experience swelling in the airway.

Spasm: Water, when suddenly inhaled, can cause a spasm in the throat. This happens in about 10 percent of all drownings. When such a spasm does not allow the lungs to fill with water, it is known as a "dry drowning."

How to Recognize Choking

Partial air exchange:

- Good—indicated by coughing forcefully by a conscious victim.
- Poor—indicated by weak, ineffective cough; high pitched noise; blue, gray, or ashen skin.

Breathing sounds which may indicate partial air exchange:

1. Snoring—tongue may be blocking airway

2. Crowing—voice box spasm

3. Wheezing—airway swelling or spasm

4. Gurgling—blood, vomit, or other liquid in airway

Complete blockage:

- Unable to speak, breathe, or cough
- Clutches neck with one or both hands (known as the "universal distress signal for choking")

Causes of Choking

The most common foods that cause choking in children include: hot dogs, candy, peanuts, and grapes. Adult choking is related to these behaviors:

- Trying to swallow large pieces of food
- Drunkenness
- Wearing dentures (false teeth)
- Eating too fast
- Eating while talking or laughing
- Walking, running, or playing with objects in mouth

Types of Foreign Body Airway Obstructions

- *Type 0:* Commonly experienced by most people; it is not life-threatening.
- *Type 1 (also known as the "lid" type):* Obstruction is on the mouth side of the epiglottis; is life-threatening.
- *Type 2 (also known as the "plug" type):* Obstruction is on the lung side of the epiglottis; is life-threatening.
- *Type 3:* Subacute choking involving a foreign body in the bronchi, but is not acutely life-threatening. Only a physician can remove (i.e., bronchoscopy or surgery).

Reasons that Some Attempts to Remove a Foreign Object Fail

- Delay in trying to resuscitate
- Incorrect techniques
- Position or extent of obstruction (such as a crayon or string from lobster or roast beef)
- Substance spread throughout airway and/or lungs (such as peanut butter)

Disease Precautions

- A concern exists about getting diseases such as HIV which results in AIDS, Hepatitis B Virus (HBV), respiratory tract infections (e.g., influenza, mononucleosis, and tuberculosis) from a CPR manikin during CPR training.
- The American Heart Association reports that CPR manikins have never been found to be responsible for any bacterial, fungal, or viral disease.

- CPR classes should follow the manikin manufacturers' recommendations on using and maintaining their manikins.
- The viral agent causing AIDS known as HIV is delicate and is inactivated in less than 10 minutes at room temperature by several kinds of disinfectants used for cleaning manikins. No evidence to date shows that HIV/AIDS is transmitted by manikin use.

Precautions During CPR Training

- Do not practice mouth-to-mouth resuscitation on a person—practice on a manikin.
- Do not practice chest compressions on a person—practice on a manikin.
- Do not practice abdominal or chest thrusts on a person.
- Follow the Centers of Disease Control manikin cleaning procedures.

Do **not** use a training manikin *if* you have:

- Sores on the hands, lips, or face (such as a cold sore)
- An upper respiratory infection (such as a cold or sore throat)
- Known positive Hepatitis B (HBV)
- Been infected by HIV or have AIDS
- An infection or recent exposure to an infectious source

Clean manikin between each student's use by:

1. Scrubbing the manikin's entire face and inside of mouth vigorously with a four-by-four-inch gauze pad saturated with 70 percent alcohol (isopropanol or ethanol);

2. Placing the wet gauze pad over the manikin's mouth and nose for at least 30 seconds; allowing manikin's face to dry.

During training, students should practice and become familiar with mouth-to-barrier devices.

Precautions During Actual CPR

- Laypersons are most likely to perform CPR in the home and will usually know the health status of the victim.
- It should be assumed that certain body fluids may have the potential to spread disease either to the victim or the rescuer.
- Transmissions of HBV and HIV infection during rescue breathing has not been documented.
- HBV-positive saliva has not been shown to be infectious. A theoretical risk of spreading HIV and HBV exists during rescue breathing if either the victim or rescuer has breaks in the skin, on or around the lips, or inside the mouth.
- The Centers for Disease Control (CDC) and the Occupational Safety and Health Administration (OSHA) constructed guidelines which include the use of latex gloves and resuscitation masks with valves capable of diverting exhaled air from contacting the rescuer.
- Rescuers should not fear getting a disease, but many may be unwilling to help a person in need because of this fear. Rescuers should learn mouth-to-barrier device (face mask or face shield) use.
- Two types of mouth-to-barrier devices exist (see Appendix C):

1. *Mask devices.* These have a one-way valve so that exhaled air does not enter the rescuer's mouth.

2. *Face shields.* These have no exhalation valve and air can leak around the shield.

- If a rescuer refuses to start rescue breathing because of fear of disease he or she should:
    1. Activate the EMS system
    2. Open the airway
    3. Give chest compressions until another rescuer arrives who will give rescue breathing

CPR Performance Mistakes

While giving rescue breathing and chest compressions, try to avoid the following mistakes.

Rescue breathing mistakes:

- Inadequate head tilt
- Failing to pinch nose shut
- Not giving slow breaths
- Failing to watch chest and listen for exhalation
- Failing to maintain tight seal around victim's mouth (and/or nose)

Chest compression mistakes:

- Pivoting at knees instead of hips (rocking motion)
- Wrong compression site
- Bending elbows
- Shoulders not above sternum (arms not vertical)
- Fingers touching chest
- Heel of bottom hand not in line with sternum
- Placing palm rather than the heel of the hand on sternum
- Lifting hands off chest between compressions (bouncing movement)
- Incorrect compression rate and/or ratio
- Jerky or jabbing compressions rather than smooth compressions

How to Remember the Basic Life Support Steps

Basic Life Support for an Adult Victim

R   Responsive?
A   Activate EMS system (usually call 9-1-1)
P   Position victim on back

A   Airway open (use head-tilt/chin-lift or jaw thrust)
B   Breathing check (look, listen, and feel for 3–5 seconds)
- If breathing and spinal injury not suspected, place in recovery position
- If not breathing, give 2 slow breaths; watch chest rise
  - If 2 breaths go in proceed to step C
  - If 2 breaths did not go in, retilt head and try 2 more breaths
  - If second 2 breaths did not go in, give 5 abdominal thrusts; perform tongue-jaw lift followed by a finger sweep; give 2 breaths, retilt head followed by 2 more breaths. Repeat thrusts, sweep, breaths sequence.
C   Circulation check (at carotid pulse for 5–10 seconds)
- If there is a pulse, but no breathing give rescue breathing (1 breath every 5–6 seconds)
- If there is no pulse, give CPR (cycles of 15 chest compressions followed by 2 breaths)

After 1 minute (4 cycles of CPR or 10–12 breaths of rescue breathing), check pulse.
- If no pulse give CPR (15:2 cycles) starting with chest compressions
- If there is a pulse but no breathing, give rescue breathing.

Basic Life Support for a Child or Infant Victim

E   Establish unresponsive
S   Send bystander, if available, to activate the EMS system (usually call 9-1-1).
P   Position victim on back

A   Airway open (use head-tilt/chin-lift or jaw thrust)
B   Breathing check (look, listen, and feel for 3–5 seconds)
- If breathing and spinal injury not suspected, place in recovery position
- If not breathing, give 2 slow breaths; watch chest rise
  - If 2 breaths go in proceed to step C
  - If 2 breaths did not go in, retilt head and try 2 more breaths
  - If second 2 breaths did not go in, then . . .
  For a child: give 5 abdominal thrusts; perform tongue-jaw lift and if object is seen perform a finger sweep; give 2 breaths, retilt head followed by 2 more breaths. Repeat thrusts, mouth check, breaths sequence
  For an infant: give 5 back blows and 5 chest thrusts; perform tongue-jaw lift and if object is seen perform a finger sweep; give 2 breaths, retilt head followed by 2 more breaths. Repeat blows, thrusts, mouth check, breaths.
C   Circulation check (at carotid pulse for 5–10 seconds)
- *For a child:* at carotid pulse
  For an infant: at brachial pulse
- If there is a pulse, but no breathing give rescue breathing (1 breath every 3 seconds)
- If there is no pulse, give CPR (cycles of 5 chest compressions followed by 1 breath)

After 1 minute (20 cycles of CPR or 20 breaths of rescue breathing), check pulse.
- If alone, activate EMS system
- If no pulse, give CPR (5:1 cycles) starting with chest compressions
- If there is a pulse but no breathing, give rescue breathing.

Basic Life Support Procedures and Techniques

Adult Rescue Breathing and CPR

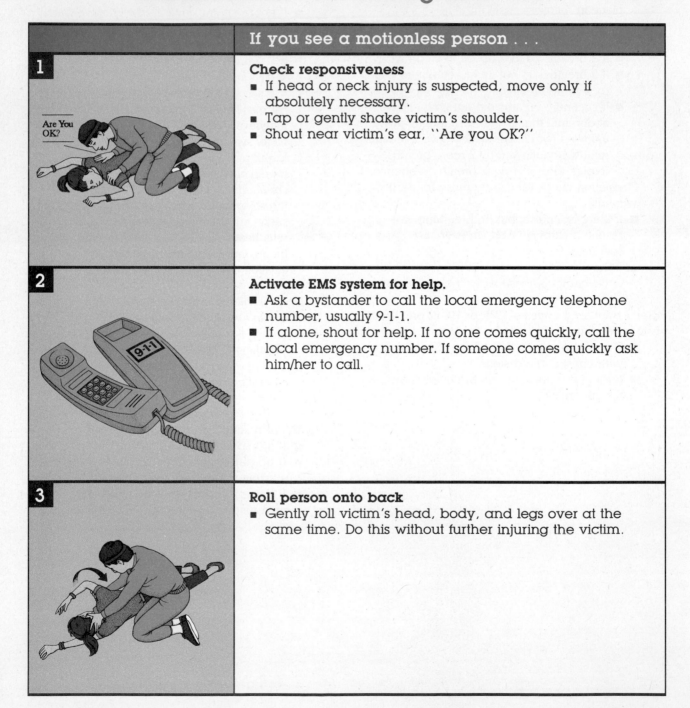

	If you see a motionless person . . .
1	**Check responsiveness** ■ If head or neck injury is suspected, move only if absolutely necessary. ■ Tap or gently shake victim's shoulder. ■ Shout near victim's ear, "Are you OK?"
2	**Activate EMS system for help.** ■ Ask a bystander to call the local emergency telephone number, usually 9-1-1. ■ If alone, shout for help. If no one comes quickly, call the local emergency number. If someone comes quickly ask him/her to call.
3	**Roll person onto back** ■ Gently roll victim's head, body, and legs over at the same time. Do this without further injuring the victim.

4

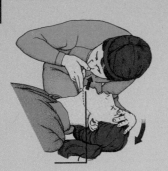

Open airway (use head-tilt/chin-lift method)
- Place hand nearest victim's head on victim's forehead and apply backward pressure to tilt head back.
- Place fingers of other hand under bony part of jaw near chin and lift. Avoid pressing on soft tissues under jaw.
- Tilt head backward without closing victim's mouth.
- Do *not* use your thumb to lift the chin.

If you suspect a neck injury
Do *not* move victim's head or neck. First try lifting chin without tilting head back. If breaths do not go in, slowly and gently bend the head back until breaths can go in.

5

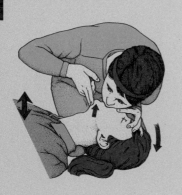

Check for breathing (take 3–5 seconds)
- Place your ear over victim's mouth and nose while keeping airway open.
- *Look* at victim's chest to check for rise and fall; *listen* and *feel* for breathing.

6

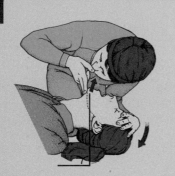

Give 2 slow breaths
- Keep head tilted back with head-tilt/chin-tilt to keep airway open.
- Pinch nose shut.
- Take a deep breath and seal your lips tightly around victim's mouth.
- Give 2 slow breaths, each lasting 1½ to 2 seconds (you should take a breath after each breath given to victim).
- Watch chest rise to see if your breaths go in.
- Allow for chest deflation after each breath.

If neither of these 2 breaths went in
Retilt the head and try 2 more breaths. If still unsuccessful, suspect choking, also known as foreign body airway obstruction (use *Unconscious Adult Foreign Body Airway Obstruction* procedures).

If you cannot use victim's mouth (e.g., injured, teeth clenched, etc.), seal your lips around victim's nose and breathe into nose. Remove your mouth to allow exhalation.

 Whenever available, use a mouth-to-barrier device. See Appendix C for details.

7

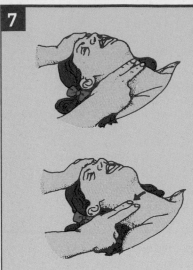

Check for pulse
- Maintain head-tilt with hand nearest head on forehead.
- Locate Adam's apple with 2 or 3 fingers of hand nearest victim's feet.
- Slide your fingers down into groove of neck on side closest to you (do not use your thumb because you may feel your own pulse).
- Feel for carotid pulse (take 5–10 seconds). Carotid artery is used because it lies close to the heart and is accessible.

8

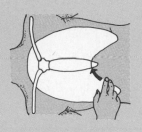

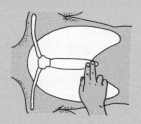

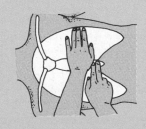

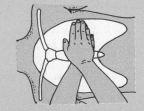

Perform rescue procedures based upon what you found:

If there is a pulse, but no breathing
Give one rescue breath (mouth-to-mouth resuscitation) every 5 to 6 seconds. Use the same techniques for rescue breathing found in Step 6 above but only give one. Every minute (10 to 12 breaths) stop and check the pulse to make sure there is a pulse. Continue until:
- Adult starts breathing on his or her own.

OR
- Trained help, such as emergency medical technicians (EMTs), arrive and relieve you.

OR
- You are completely exhausted.

If there is no pulse, give CPR
- Find hand position

   1. Use your fingers to slide up rib cage edge nearest you to notch at the end of sternum.

   2. Place your middle finger on or in the notch and index finger next to it.

   3. Put heel of other hand (one closest to victim's head) on sternum next to index finger.

   4. Remove hand from notch and put it on top of hand on chest.

   5. Interlace, hold, or extend fingers up

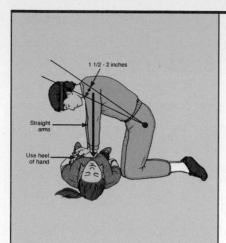

- Do 15 compressions.

    1. Place your shoulders directly over your hands on the chest.

    2. Keep arms straight and elbows locked.

    3. Push sternum straight down 1½ to 2 inches.

    4. Do 15 compressions at 80 per minute. Count as you push down: "one and, two and, three and, four and, five and, six and, seven and . . . . fifteen and."

    5. Push smoothly; do not jerk or jab; do not stop at the top or at the bottom.

    6. When pushing, bend from your hips, not knees.

    7. Keep fingers pointing across victim's chest, away from you.

- Give 2 slow breaths
- Complete four cycles of 15 compressions and two breaths (takes about 1 minute) and check the pulse. *If there is no pulse,* restart CPR with chest compressions. Recheck the pulse every few minutes. *If there is a pulse,* give rescue breathing.
- Give CPR or rescue breathing until:
Victim revives.
OR
Trained help, such as emergency medical technicians (EMTs), arrives and relieves you.
OR
You are completely exhausted.

Conscious Adult Foreign Body Airway Obstruction (Choking)

	If person is conscious and cannot speak, breathe, or cough . . .
1	**Give up to 5 abdominal thrusts** (Heimlich maneuver): ■ Stand behind the victim. ■ Wrap your arms around victim's waist. (Do not allow your forearms to touch the ribs.) ■ Make a fist with 1 hand and place the thumb side just above victim's navel and well below the tip of the sternum. ■ Grasp fist with your other hand. ■ Press fist into victim's abdomen with 5 quick upward thrusts. ■ Each thrust should be a separate and distinct effort to dislodge the object. After every 5 abdominal thrusts, check the victim and your technique. Note: For advanced pregnant women and obese victims consider using chest thrusts.
2	**Repeat cycles of up to 5 abdominal thrusts until:** ■ Victim coughs up object. OR ■ Victim starts to breathe or coughs forcefully. OR ■ Victim becomes unconscious (activate EMS and start methods for an unconscious victim with a finger sweep first). OR ■ You are relieved by EMS or other trained person. Reassess victim and your technique after every 5 thrusts.

Unconscious Adult Foreign Body Airway Obstruction (Choking)

	If person is unconscious and breaths have not gone in . . .
1	**Give up to 5 abdominal thrusts** (Heimlich maneuver): ■ Straddle victim's thighs. ■ Put heel of one hand against middle of victim's abdomen slightly above navel and well below sternum's notch (fingers of hand should point toward victim's head). ■ Put other hand directly on top of first hand. ■ Press inward and upward using both hands with up to 5 quick abdominal thrusts. ■ Each thrust should be distinct and a real attempt made to relieve the airway obstruction. Keep heel of hand in contact with abdomen between abdominal thrusts. Note: For advanced pregnant women and obese victims consider using chest thrusts.
2	**Perform finger sweep** ■ Use only on an unconscious victim. On a conscious victim, it may cause gagging or vomiting. ■ Use your thumb and fingers to grasp victim's jaw and tongue and lift upward to pull tongue away from back of throat and away from foreign object. ■ If unable to open mouth to perform the tongue-jaw lift, use the crossed-finger method by crossing the index finger and thumb and pushing the teeth apart. ■ With index finger of your other hand, slide finger down along the inside of one cheek deeply into mouth and use a hooking action across to other cheek to dislodge foreign object. ■ If foreign body comes within reach, grab and remove it. Do not force object deeper.
3	**If the above steps are unsuccessful** Cycle through the following steps in rapid sequence until the object is expelled or EMS arrives: ■ Give 2 rescue breaths. If unsuccessful, retilt head and try 2 more breaths. ■ Do up to 5 abdominal thrusts. ■ Do a finger sweep.

Adult Basic Life Support
Proficiency Checklist

S = self-check / P = partner check / I = instructor check

Adult Rescue Breathing

	S	P	I
1. Check responsiveness	☐	☐	☐
2. Activate EMS	☐	☐	☐
3. Roll victim onto back	☐	☐	☐
4. Airway open	☐	☐	☐
5. Breathing check	☐	☐	☐
6. 2 slow breaths	☐	☐	☐
7. Check pulse at carotid	☐	☐	☐
8. Rescue breathing (1 every 5 to 6 seconds)	☐	☐	☐
9. Recheck pulse and breathing after first minute then every few minutes	☐	☐	☐

Adult One-Rescuer CPR

	S	P	I
1. Check responsiveness	☐	☐	☐
2. Activate EMS	☐	☐	☐
3. Roll victim onto back	☐	☐	☐
4. Airway open	☐	☐	☐
5. Breathing check	☐	☐	☐
6. 2 slow breaths	☐	☐	☐
7. Check pulse at carotid	☐	☐	☐
8. Hand position	☐	☐	☐
9. 15 compressions	☐	☐	☐
10. 2 slow breaths	☐	☐	☐
11. Continue CPR (3 more cycles for total of 4)	☐	☐	☐
12. Recheck pulse	☐	☐	☐
13. Continue CPR (start with compressions)	☐	☐	☐
14. Recheck pulse after first minute then every few minutes	☐	☐	☐

Conscious Adult Choking Management

	S	P	I
1. Recognize choking	☐	☐	☐
2. Up to 5 abdominal thrusts	☐	☐	☐
3. Reassess	☐	☐	☐
4. Repeat cycles of up to 5 thrusts; reassess after each cycle	☐	☐	☐

Unconscious Adult Choking Management

	S	P	I
1. Check responsiveness	☐	☐	☐
2. Activate EMS	☐	☐	☐
3. Roll victim onto back	☐	☐	☐
4. Airway open	☐	☐	☐
5. Breathing check	☐	☐	☐
6. Try 2 slow breaths. If unsuccessful, retilt head and try 2 more	☐	☐	☐
7. Up to 5 abdominal thrusts	☐	☐	☐
8. Finger sweep	☐	☐	☐
9. Try 2 slow breaths. If unsuccessful, retilt head and try 2 more	☐	☐	☐
10. Repeat "thrusts, sweep, breaths" sequence	☐	☐	☐

Differences Between Adult and Child (1–8 years) Basic Life Support

IF child . . .	THEN . . .
is **not** responsive and rescuer is alone	**activate EMS system after 1 minute of resuscitation** (in adults, activate EMS system immediately after determining unresponsiveness)
is **not** breathing, but has a pulse	▪ give **1 to 1½ seconds breaths** (in adults give 1½ to 2 seconds breaths) ▪ give **1 breath every 3 seconds** (in adults give 1 breath every 5 to 6 seconds)
does **not** have a pulse	▪ after locating the tip of the breastbone, lift your fingers off and put heel of the **same hand** on breastbone immediately above where index finger was (adult requires one hand to locate and the other hand placed next to it) ▪ give **chest compressions with 1 hand** (nearest feet) while keeping other hand on child's forehead (adult requires 2 hands on victim's chest for compressions) ▪ **compress breastbone 1 to 1½ inches** (adults require 1½ to 2 inches) ▪ give **one breath after every 5 chest compressions** (one-rescuer adult CPR requires 2 breaths after every 15 compressions)
has a foreign body airway obstruction (choking), and after giving up to 5 abdominal thrusts (Heimlich maneuver), the airway still remains obstructed	look into mouth; **remove foreign body only if seen with finger sweep—do not perform blind finger sweeps** (in an adult, you can perform blind finger sweeps)

Infant (under 1 year) Rescue Breathing and CPR

Check responsiveness
- If head or neck injury is suspected, move only if absolutely necessary.
- Tap or gently shake infant's shoulder.

Send bystander, if available, to activate the EMS system. If alone, give rescue breathing or CPR for one minute before activating the EMS system.

Roll infant onto back
Gently roll infant's head, body, and legs over at the same time (avoid twisting).

4

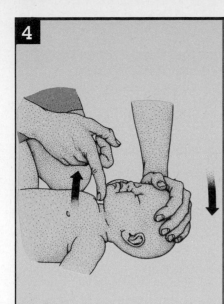

Open airway (use head-tilt/chin-lift method)
- Place hand nearest infant's head on infant's forehead and apply backward pressure to tilt head back (known as the "sniffing" or neutral position).
- Place fingers of other hand under bony part of jaw near chin and lift. Avoid pressing on soft tissues under jaw.
- Tilt head backward without closing infant's mouth.
- Do not use your thumb to lift the chin.

If you suspect a neck injury
Do not move infant's head or neck. First try lifting chin without tilting head back. If breaths do not go in, slowly and gently bend the head back until breaths can go in.

5

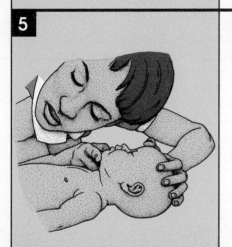

Check for breathing (take 3–5 seconds)
- Place your ear over infant's mouth and nose while keeping airway open.
- Look at infant's chest to check for rise and fall; listen and feel for breathing.

6

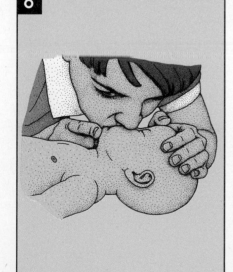

Give 2 slow breaths
- Keep head tilted back with head-tilt/chin-lift to keep airway open
- With your mouth make a seal over infant's mouth and nose.
- Give 2 slow breaths, each lasting 1 to 1½ seconds (you should take a breath after each breath given).
- Watch chest rise to see if your breaths go in.
- Allow for chest deflation after each breath.

If neither of these 2 breaths went in
Retilt the head and try 2 more breaths. If still unsuccessful, suspect choking, also known as foreign body airway obstruction (refer to the Unconscious Infant Foreign Body Airway Obstruction section).

 Whenever available, use a mouth-to-barrier device. See Appendix C for details.

7

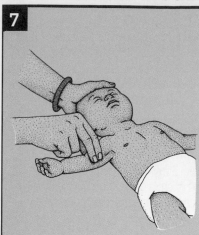

Check for pulse
- Maintain head-tilt with hand nearest head on forehead.
- Feel for pulse located on the inside of the upper arm between the elbow and armpit (known as the brachial).
- Press gently with 2 fingers on inside of arm closest to you.
- Place thumb of same hand on outside of infant's upper arm.

8

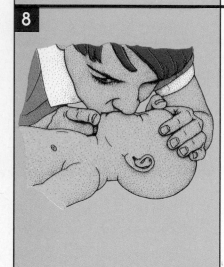

Perform rescue procedures based upon your pulse check.

If there is a pulse
Give rescue breaths (mouth-to-mouth resuscitation) every 3 seconds. Use the same techniques for rescue breathing found in Step 6 above but only give one breath. Every minute (20 breaths) stop and check the pulse to make sure there is a pulse. Continue until:
- Infant starts breathing on his or her own.

OR
- Trained help, such as emergency medical technicians (EMTs), arrive and relieve you.

OR
- You are completely exhausted.

 Whenever available, use a mouth-to-barrier device. See Appendix C for details.

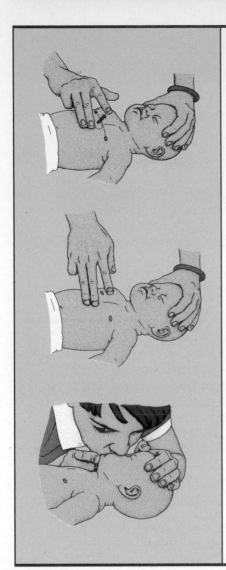

If there is no pulse, give CPR:

- Locate fingers' position

    1. Maintain head-tilt

    2. Imagine a line connecting the nipples

    3. Place 3 fingers on sternum with index finger touching but below imaginary nipple line.

    4. Raise your index finger and use other 2 fingers for compression. If you feel the notch at the end of the sternum, move your fingers up a little.

- Give 5 compressions

    1. Do 5 chest compressions at rate of 100 per minute or count as you push down, "one, two, three, four, five."

    2. Press sternum ½ to 1 inch or about ⅓ to ½ of the depth of the chest.

    3. Keep fingers pointing across the infant's chest away from you. Keep fingers in contact with infant's chest.

    4. Maintain head-tilt with hand nearest head on forehead.

- Give 1 breath
- Complete 20 cycles of 5 compressions and 1 breath (takes about 1 minute) and check the pulse. If rescuer is alone, activate the EMS system. If there is no pulse, restart CPR with chest compressions. Recheck the pulse every few minutes. If there is a pulse, give rescue breathing.
- Give CPR until:

    Infant revives.

    OR

    Trained help, such as emergency medical technicians (EMTs), arrives and relieves you.

    OR

    You are completely exhausted.

 Whenever available, use a mouth-to-barrier device. See Appendix C for details.

Conscious Infant Foreign Body Airway Obstruction (Choking)

	If infant is conscious and cannot cough, cry, or breathe . . .
1	**Give up to 5 back blows** ■ Hold infant's head and neck with 1 hand by firmly holding infant's jaw between your thumb and fingers. ■ Lay infant face down over your forearm with head lower than his/her chest. Brace your forearm and infant against your thigh. ■ Give up to 5 distinct and separate back blows between shoulder blades with the heel of your hand.
2	**Give up to 5 chest thrusts** ■ Support the back of infant's head. ■ Sandwich infant between your hands and arms, turn on back, with head lower than his/her chest. Small rescuers may need to support infant on their lap. ■ Imagine a line connecting infant's nipples. ■ Place 3 fingers on sternum with your ring finger next to imaginary nipple line on the infant's feet side. ■ Lift your ring finger off chest. If you feel the notch at the end of the sternum, move your fingers up a little. ■ Give up to 5 separate and distinct thrusts with index and middle fingers on sternum in a manner similar to CPR chest compressions, but at a slower rate. ■ Keep fingers in contact with chest between chest thrusts.

3	**Repeat**
	  1. Up to 5 back blows
	  2. Up to 5 chest thrusts until:
	    ■ infant becomes unconscious, or
	    ■ object is expelled and infant begins to breathe or coughs forcefully

Unconscious Infant with Foreign Body Airway Obstruction (Choking)

If infant is motionless . . .

1

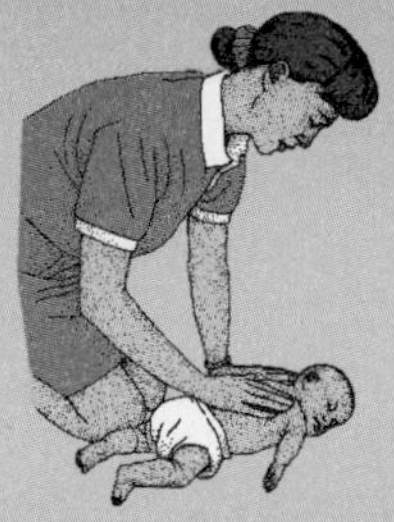

Check responsiveness
- If head or neck injury is suspected, move only if absolutely necessary.
- Tap or gently shake infant's shoulder.

2

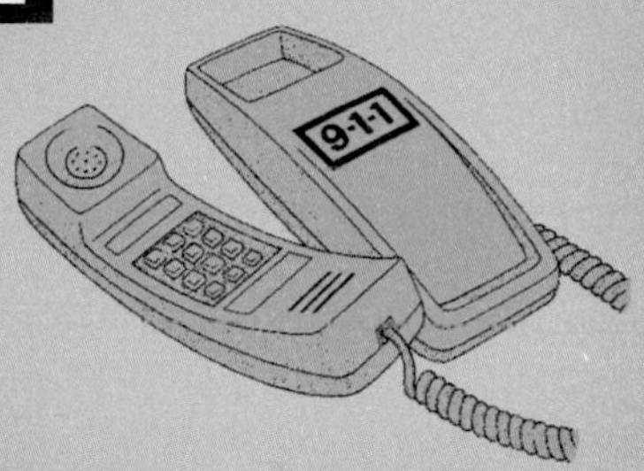

Send bystander, if available, to activate the EMS system. If alone, resuscitate for one minute before activating the EMS system.

3

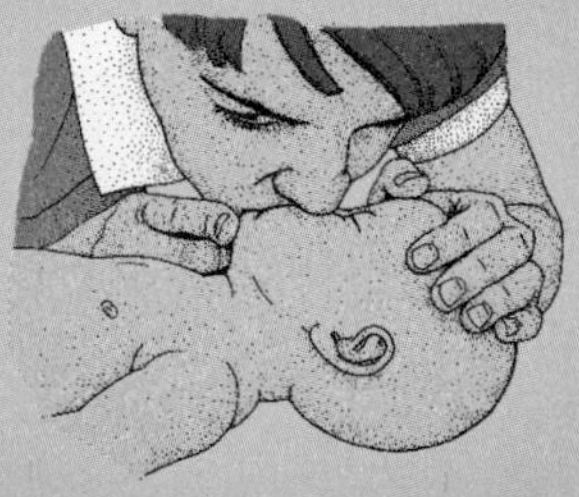

Give 2 slow breaths
- Open the airway with head-tilt/chin-lift.
- Seal your mouth over infant's mouth and nose.
- Give 2 slow breaths (1 to 1½ seconds each)

If first 2 breaths do not go in, retilt the head and try 2 more slow breaths.

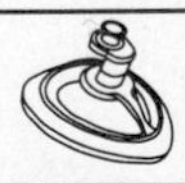

Whenever available, use a mouth-to-barrier device. See Appendix C for details.

4

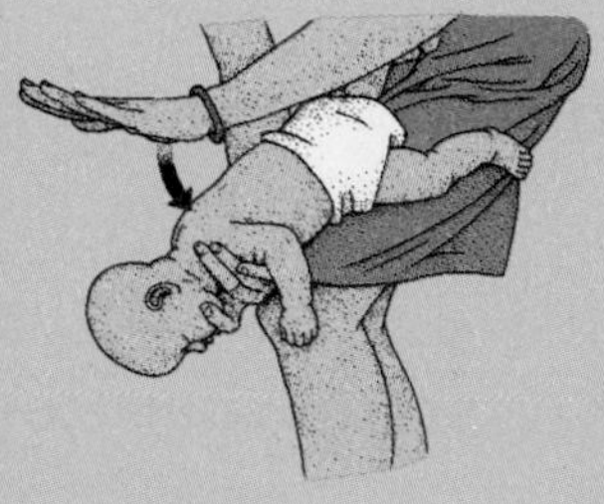

Give up to 5 back blows
- Hold infant's head and neck with 1 hand by firmly holding infant's jaw between your thumb and fingers.
- Lay infant face down over your forearm with head lower than his/her chest. Brace your forearm and infant against your thigh.
- Give up to 5 distinct and separate back blows between shoulder blades with the heel of your hand.

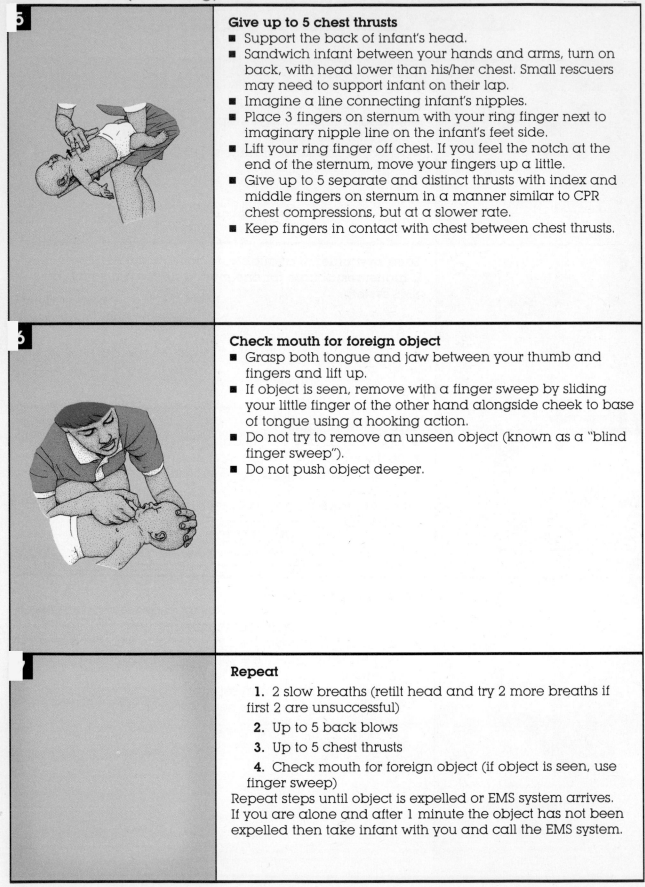

5

Give up to 5 chest thrusts

- Support the back of infant's head.
- Sandwich infant between your hands and arms, turn on back, with head lower than his/her chest. Small rescuers may need to support infant on their lap.
- Imagine a line connecting infant's nipples.
- Place 3 fingers on sternum with your ring finger next to imaginary nipple line on the infant's feet side.
- Lift your ring finger off chest. If you feel the notch at the end of the sternum, move your fingers up a little.
- Give up to 5 separate and distinct thrusts with index and middle fingers on sternum in a manner similar to CPR chest compressions, but at a slower rate.
- Keep fingers in contact with chest between chest thrusts.

6

Check mouth for foreign object

- Grasp both tongue and jaw between your thumb and fingers and lift up.
- If object is seen, remove with a finger sweep by sliding your little finger of the other hand alongside cheek to base of tongue using a hooking action.
- Do not try to remove an unseen object (known as a "blind finger sweep").
- Do not push object deeper.

7

Repeat

1. 2 slow breaths (retilt head and try 2 more breaths if first 2 are unsuccessful)

2. Up to 5 back blows

3. Up to 5 chest thrusts

4. Check mouth for foreign object (if object is seen, use finger sweep)

Repeat steps until object is expelled or EMS system arrives. If you are alone and after 1 minute the object has not been expelled then take infant with you and call the EMS system.

Infant Basic Life Support
Proficiency Checklist

S = self-check / P = partner check / I = instructor check

Infant Rescue Breathing

	S	P	I
1. Check responsiveness	☐	☐	☐
2. Send a bystander, if available, to call EMS	☐	☐	☐
3. Roll infant onto back	☐	☐	☐
4. **A**irway open	☐	☐	☐
5. **B**reathing check	☐	☐	☐
6. 2 slow breaths	☐	☐	☐
7. **C**heck pulse at brachial	☐	☐	☐
8. Rescue breathing (1 every 3 seconds)	☐	☐	☐
9. Call EMS after 1 minute	☐	☐	☐
10 Recheck pulse and breathing after first minute then every few minutes	☐	☐	☐

Infant CPR

	S	P	I
1. Check responsiveness	☐	☐	☐
2. Send a bystander, if available, to call EMS	☐	☐	☐
3. Roll infant onto back	☐	☐	☐
4. **A**irway open	☐	☐	☐
5. **B**reathing check	☐	☐	☐
6. 2 slow breaths	☐	☐	☐
7. **C**heck pulse at brachial	☐	☐	☐
8. Find fingers' position	☐	☐	☐
9. 5 chest compressions	☐	☐	☐
10. 1 slow breath	☐	☐	☐
11. Continue CPR for 1 minute (19 more cycles for total of 20)	☐	☐	☐
12. Call EMS	☐	☐	☐
13. Recheck pulse	☐	☐	☐
14. Continue CPR (start with compressions)	☐	☐	☐
15. Recheck pulse after first minute then every few minutes	☐	☐	☐

Conscious Infant Choking Management

	S	P	I
1. Recognize choking.	☐	☐	☐
2. Up to 5 back blows (head and face down)	☐	☐	☐
3. Up to 5 chest thrusts (head down with face up)	☐	☐	☐
4. Repeat steps #2 and #3	☐	☐	☐

Unconscious Infant Choking Management

	S	P	I
1. Check responsiveness	☐	☐	☐
2. Send a bystander, if available, to call EMS	☐	☐	☐
3. Roll infant onto back	☐	☐	☐
4. **A**irway open	☐	☐	☐
5. **B**reathing check	☐	☐	☐
6. Try 2 slow breaths (retilt head and try 2 more if unsuccessful)	☐	☐	☐
7. Up to 5 back blows (head and face down)	☐	☐	☐
8. Up to 5 chest thrusts (head down and face up)	☐	☐	☐
9. Check mouth for foreign object (finger sweep only if object seen)	☐	☐	☐
10. Try 2 slow breaths (if unsuccessful, retilt head and try 2 more)	☐	☐	☐
11. Repeat "blows, thrusts, mouth check, breaths"	☐	☐	☐

CPR Review

ITEM	INFANT (0–1 year)	CHILD (1–8 years)	ADULT (>8 years)
How to open airway?	Head-tilt/chin-lift	Head-tilt/chin-lift	Head-tilt/chin-lift
How to check breathing?	Look at chest and listen and feel for air (3–5 seconds)	Look at chest and listen and feel for air (3–5 seconds)	Look at chest and listen and feel for air (3–5 seconds)
What kinds of breaths?	Slow, make chest rise and fall	Slow, make chest rise and fall	Slow, make chest rise and fall
Where to check pulse?	Brachial artery (5–10 seconds)	Carotid artery (5–10 seconds)	Carotid artery (5–10 seconds)
Hand position for chest compressions?	1 finger's width below imaginary line between nipples	1 finger's width above tip of sternum	1 finger's width above tip of sternum
Compress with?	2 fingers	Heel of 1 hand	Heels of 2 hands, one hand on top of the other
Compression depth?	½–1 inch	1–1½ inches	1½–2 inches
Compression rate?	100 per minute	100 per minute	80–100 per minute
Compression:breath ratio?	5:1	5:1	15:2
How to count for compression rate?	1,2,3,4,5, breathe	1 and 2 and 3 and 4 and 5 and breathe	1 and 2 and 3 and 4 and 5 and 6 and . . . 15 and breathe, breathe
How often to reassess?	After the first minute, then every few minutes	After the first minute, then every few minutes	After the first minute, then every few minutes
After reassessment, resume CPR with?	Compressions	Compressions	Compressions
How often to give only breaths during rescue breathing?	Every 3 seconds	Every 3 seconds	Every 5 seconds

Name _____ Course _____ Date _____

■ ACTIVITY 1 ■ Adult Resuscitation

Choose the best answer.

1. ____ Are chest compressions likely to work if the victim is on a soft surface?
   A. Yes, a soft surface is okay.
   B. No, the surface should be hard.

2. ____ When you tip the head with the chin lift, where do you place your fingertips?
   A. Under the soft part of the throat near the chin
   B. Under the bony part of the jaw near the chin

3. ____ Which is the safer way to open the airway of a person who may have neck or back injuries?
   A. Push the jaw forward from the corners.
   B. Tip the head very gently, part way back.

4. ____ How should you check for stopped breathing?
   A. Look at the chest; listen and feel for air coming out of the mouth.
   B. Look at the pupils of the eyes.
   C. Check the pulse.

5. ____ When you give breaths to an adult, the breaths should be:
   A. Slow
   B. Fast

6. ____ Before deciding whether to give CPR, check the victim's pulse for:
   A. 1–3 seconds   B. 3–5 seconds
   C. 5–10 seconds   D. 1–20 seconds

7. ____ To find where to push on the chest for chest compressions, you should measure up:
   A. Two hand-widths from the navel.
   B. One finger-width from the middle finger on the sternum's tip.

8. ____ Give chest compressions:
   A. With a quick jerk
   B. Smoothly and regularly

9. ____ Push on a victim's chest:
   A. At an angle
   B. Straight down

10. ____ Compress an adult's chest at least:
    A. ½ to 1 inch
    B. 1½ to 2 inches

11. ____ In one-rescuer CPR, give chest compressions to an adult at the rate, per minute, of:
    A. 100
    B. 80
    C. 60
    D. 40

12. ____ What is the pattern of compressions and breaths in one-rescuer CPR for an adult victim?
    A. 15 compressions, 2 breaths
    B. 15 compressions, 1 breath
    C. 5 compressions, 2 breaths
    D. 5 compressions, 1 breath

■ ACTIVITY 2 ■ Adult Choking

Choose the best answer.

1. ____ An adult victim is coughing forcefully. Should you give back blows and thrusts?
   A. Yes
   B. No

2. ____ A person is coughing weakly and making wheezing noises. You should:
   A. Give abdominal thrusts.
   B. Let the person alone and watch closely.

3. ____ A victim who seems to be choking *can* speak. Should you give abdominal thrusts?
   A. Yes
   B. No

4. ____ A conscious person is coughing forcefully, trying to dislodge an object. Then the person stops coughing and cannot speak. You should:
   A. Give abdominal thrusts.
   B. Let the person alone and watch closely.

5. ____ When you give abdominal thrusts to a conscious victim, what part of your fist do you place against the victim?
   A. The palm side
   B. The little finger side
   C. The thumb side
6. ____ Give abdominal thrusts quickly:
   A. Inward and upward
   B. Straight back
7. ____ Where do you place your fist to give abdominal thrusts?
   A. Over the breastbone
   B. Slightly above the navel
   C. Below the navel

8. ____ To give abdominal thrusts to a victim who is lying down, place the heel of one hand:
   A. Slightly above the navel
   B. On the edge of the breastbone
   C. Below the navel
9. ____ For a victim who is obese or in advanced pregnancy, it is better to give:
   A. Abdominal thrusts
   B. Chest thrusts

■ ACTIVITY 3 ■ Child and Infant Resuscitation

Choose the best answer.

1. ____ How should you check for stopped breathing?
   A. Look at the chest; listen and feel for air coming out of the mouth.
   B. Look at the pupils of the eyes.
   C. Check the pulse.
2. ____ If your amount of breath is enough:
   A. The stomach will form a pouch.
   B. The chest will rise.
   C. Your air backs up against incoming air.
3. ____ Check a baby's pulse at the:
   A. Middle of the upper arm
   B. Wrist
   C. Neck
4. ____ To give a baby chest compressions use:
   A. 2 or 3 fingers
   B. The heel of one hand
5. ____ Push on the chest of a child or baby one finger-width:
   A. Above nipple line
   B. Below nipple line
   C. Above xiphoid notch

6. ____ How far should you compress a baby's chest?
   A. 1½ to 2 inches
   B. ½ to 1 inch
7. ____ Give a baby chest compressions at the rate per minute, of:
   A. 100
   B. 80
   C. 60
8. ____ Give babies and children:
   A. 15 compressions, 2 breaths
   B. 5 compressions, 2 breaths
   C. 15 compressions, 1 breath
   D. 5 compressions, 1 breath
9. ____ When giving chest compressions to a child, use:
   A. 2 or 3 fingers or heel of one hand
   B. The heel of one hand and the other hand on top

■ ACTIVITY 4 ■ Child and Infant Choking

Choose the best answer.

1. ____ You believe a baby has an object caught in its airway; it cannot cough or cry. What do you do first?
   A. Let it alone and watch closely.
   B. Give abdominal thrusts.
   C. Give chest thrusts.
   D. Give back blows.

2. ____ Use your finger to remove an object from an unconscious baby or child's mouth:
   A. Whenever back blows and chest thrusts fail
   B. Only if you see the object

Shock

■ **Hypovolemic Shock** ■ **Fainting** ■ **Severe Allergic Reaction** ■

Many injuries involve some degree of shock. Shock occurs when the circulatory system fails to deliver oxygenated blood to every part of the body.

Several types of shock exist; first aiders usually concern themselves mainly with these three types: hypovolemic, fainting, and anaphylactic (better known as severe allergic reaction).

Hypovolemic

Hypovolemic shock results from blood or fluid loss. If related to blood loss it is best known as hemorrhagic shock.

Signs and Symptoms

- Rapid breathing and pulse
- Pale or bluish skin, nailbed, and lips
- Slow capillary filling time
- Cool and wet (clammy) skin
- Heavy sweating
- Dilated (enlarged) pupils
- Dull, sunken look to the eyes
- Thirst

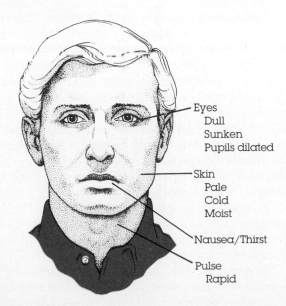

Eyes
Dull
Sunken
Pupils dilated

Skin
Pale
Cold
Moist

Nausea/Thirst

Pulse
Rapid

Signs and symptoms of shock

- Nausea and vomiting
- Loss of consciousness in severe shock

First Aid

Even if signs and symptoms have not appeared in a severely injured victim, treat for shock. **First aiders can prevent shock; they cannot reverse it**.

- Care for life-threatening injuries and other severe injuries.
- Elevate the legs 8–12 inches unless the injury makes this impossible or unless it is not advised because of chest injuries, unconsciousness, etc. Elevating the legs allows the blood to be returned to the heart more readily. Do *not* raise the legs more than 12 inches since it affects the victim's breathing by having the abdominal organs push up against the diaphragm. Do *not* lift the foot of a bed or stretcher because breathing will be affected.
- Keep the victim on his or her back. Exceptions are:

   1. Those with head injuries or stroke victims who should have their heads slightly raised if no spine injury is suspected.

   2. Those with breathing difficulties, chest injuries, or a heart attack should be in a semi-sitting position. This helps breathing.

   3. An unconscious, semiconscious, or vomiting victim should lie on his or her side.

- Prevent body heat loss by putting blankets under and over the victim. Do *not* attempt to warm the victim unless he or she is hypothermic.
- Do *not* give the victim anything to eat or drink. It could cause nausea and vomiting, which could be inhaled.
- Handle the victim very gently.

Fainting

Fainting involves a sudden, temporary loss of consciousness. It occurs when the brain's blood flow is interrupted. Numerous causes account for the interrupted blood flow.

Signs and Symptoms

Fainting may occur suddenly or may be preceded by warning signs including any or all of the following:

- Dizziness
- Seeing spots
- Nausea
- Paleness
- Sweating

First Aid

When a person appears on the verge of fainting:

- Prevent the person from falling.
- Have the person lie down and elevate the legs 8–12 inches.

If fainting has occurred or if fainting is anticipated:

- Lay the victim down and elevate the legs 8–12 inches.
- If vomiting begins, turn the person on the side to keep the airway open and clear.
- Loosen tight clothing.
- If the victim has fallen, look for injuries.
- Wet a cloth with cool water and wipe the person's forehead and face.
- Do *not* splash or pour water on the victim's face.
- Do *not* use smelling salts or ammonia.
- Do *not* slap the victim's face as an attempt to revive him or her.
- Do *not* give the victim anything to drink until fully recovered.

Most fainting cases are not serious and the victim regains consciousness quickly. However, seek medical attention if the victim:

- Is over 40 years old
- Has had repeated attacks of unconsciousness
- Does not waken within four or five minutes
- Loses consciousness while sitting or lying down
- Faints for no apparent reason

Severe Allergic Reaction (Anaphylactic Shock)

Allergies are usually thought of as causing rashes, itching, or some other short-term discomfort that disappears when the offending agent is removed from contact with the allergic person. There is, however, a more powerful reaction to substances ordinarily eaten or injected called anaphylactic shock, which can occur within minutes or even seconds. Such a reaction can cause death if not treated immediately.

Eating of certain foods, such as nuts or shellfish, or using some medications or drugs, such as oral penicillin, can cause severe reactions in sensitive persons.

The sting of a honeybee, wasp, yellow jacket, or hornet can cause very severe, immediate reactions in those allergic to the injected toxin. About one percent of the population is severely sensitive to insect stings.

The injection of a drug such as penicillin or a tetanus antitoxin may cause an immediate severe reaction.

The severe allergic response (anaphylactic shock) is triggered by contact with a substance that the individual has previously encountered and the body has identified as an enemy, causing the development of antibodies called IgE. The antibodies, or body defenders, later come in contact with the offending substance and release chemicals (e.g., histamine) that attack the lungs, blood vessels, intestines, and skin.

It is a life-threatening situation! About 60–80% of anaphylactic deaths are caused by an inability to breathe because swollen airway passages obstruct airflow to the lungs. The second most common cause of anaphylactic deaths—about 24%—is shock, brought on by insufficient blood circulating through the body.

Signs and Symptoms

One or all of these signs and symptoms may appear:

- Coughing, sneezing, or wheezing
- Difficult breathing
- Tightness and swelling in the throat
- Tightness in the chest
- Severe itching, burning, rash, or hives on the skin
- Swollen face, tongue, mouth
- Nausea and vomiting
- Dizziness
- Abdominal cramps
- Blueness (cyanosis) around the lips and mouth

First Aid

This is a true emergency! Seek medical attention for the victim.

Epinephrine is the emergency treatment of severe allergic reactions (anaphylaxis) to insect stings or bites, foods, drugs, and other allergens. For such emergency situations, an epinephrine injection kit prescribed by a physician and carried by the victim is necessary. The epinephrine is intended to be immediately self-administered by a person with a history of anaphylactic reaction. Despite any concerns, epinephrine is essential for the treatment of anaphylaxis. First aiders can assist the victim to administer his or her own epinephrine. First aiders do not have access to epinephrine except through a victim's kit.

Follow the instructions included in the kit. The kit's epinephrine is in a syringe and ready for injection. Keep checking the victim after the injection since a second injection may be needed.

In some cases cardiopulmonary resuscitation (CPR) is required. It is essential that the offending substance be identified because each anaphylactic response may be more severe than the previous one.

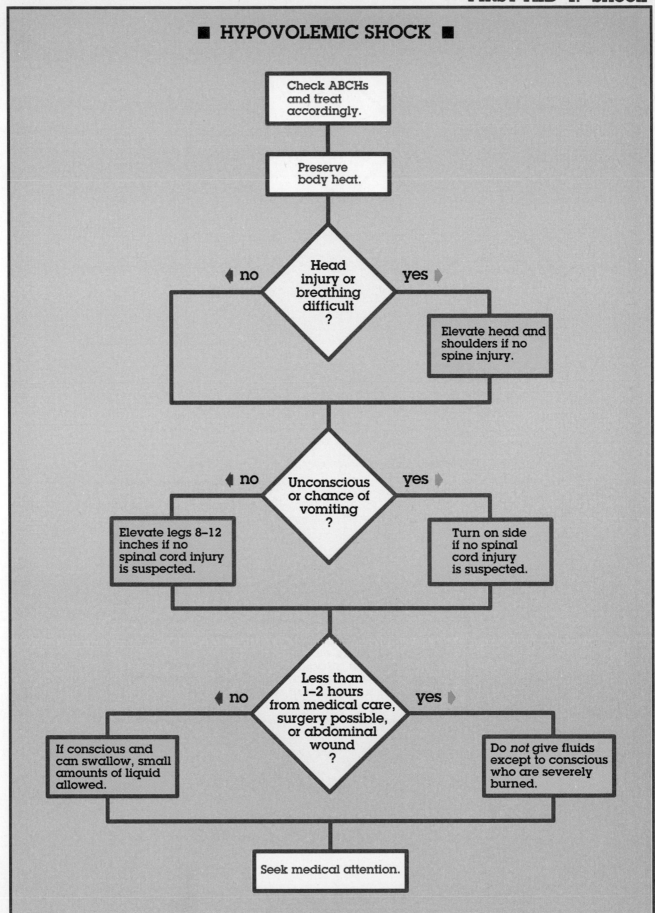

■ HYPOVOLEMIC SHOCK ■

Check ABCHs and treat accordingly.

Preserve body heat.

Head injury or breathing difficult ?

no ◄   yes ►

Elevate head and shoulders if no spine injury.

Unconscious or chance of vomiting ?

no ◄   yes ►

Elevate legs 8–12 inches if no spinal cord injury is suspected.

Turn on side if no spinal cord injury is suspected.

Less than 1–2 hours from medical care, surgery possible, or abdominal wound ?

no ◄   yes ►

If conscious and can swallow, small amounts of liquid allowed.

Do *not* give fluids except to conscious who are severely burned.

Seek medical attention.

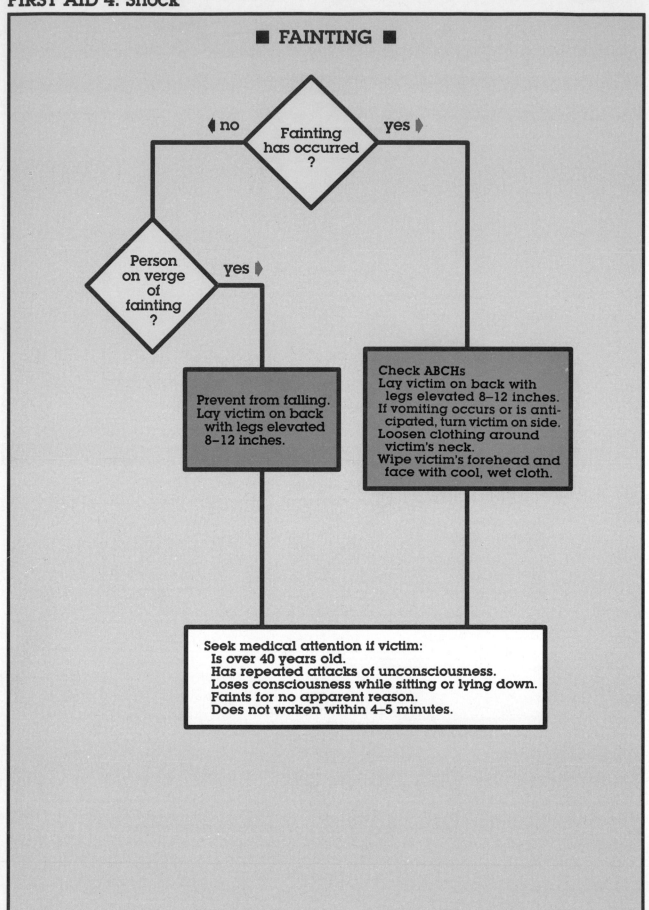

■ **FAINTING** ■

Fainting has occurred ?

← no   yes ▶

Person on verge of fainting ?

yes ▶

Prevent from falling. Lay victim on back with legs elevated 8–12 inches.

**Check ABCHs
Lay victim on back with legs elevated 8–12 inches.
If vomiting occurs or is anticipated, turn victim on side.
Loosen clothing around victim's neck.
Wipe victim's forehead and face with cool, wet cloth.**

**Seek medical attention if victim:
Is over 40 years old.
Has repeated attacks of unconsciousness.
Loses consciousness while sitting or lying down.
Faints for no apparent reason.
Does not waken within 4–5 minutes.**

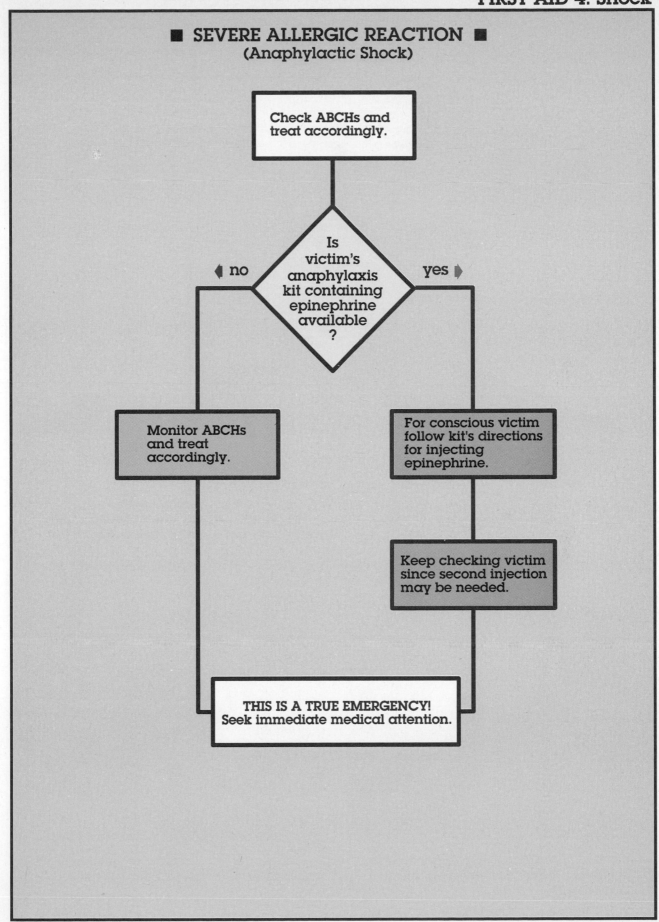

■ SEVERE ALLERGIC REACTION ■
(Anaphylactic Shock)

Check ABCHs and treat accordingly.

Is victim's anaphylaxis kit containing epinephrine available?

◀ no

yes ▶

Monitor ABCHs and treat accordingly.

For conscious victim follow kit's directions for injecting epinephrine.

Keep checking victim since second injection may be needed.

THIS IS A TRUE EMERGENCY!
Seek immediate medical attention.

SKILL SCAN: Positioning the Shock Victim

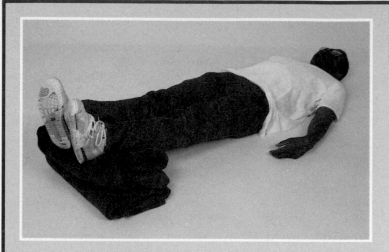

Usual shock position. Elevate the legs 8-12 inches. Do not lift the foot of bed or stretcher.

EXCEPTIONS:

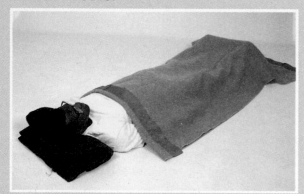

Elevate the head for injuries or stroke.

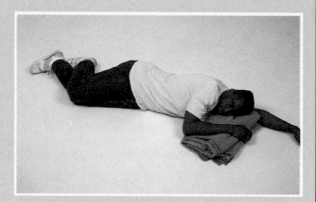

Lay an unconcious, semiconcious, or vomiting victim on his or her side.

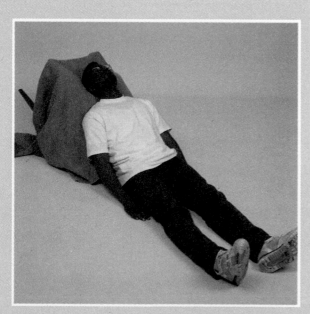

Use a semisitting position for those with breathing difficulties, chest injuries, or a heart attack.

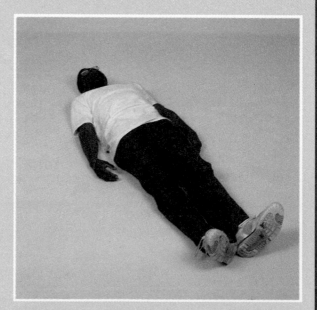

Keep victim flat if a neck or spine injury is suspected or victim has leg fractures.

■ ACTIVITY 1 ■
Hypovolemic Shock

Mark each statement true (T) or false (F).

1. ____ Shock results when parts of the body do not receive enough blood.

2. ____ Shock is a concern only in life-threatening injuries.

3. ____ People's lives can be threatened by shock.

Complete the following statement.

When a person experiences shock, usually the

1. ____ **A.** skin is pale/bluish.
   B. skin is red.

2. ____ **A.** skin is dry.
   B. skin is moist.

3. ____ **A.** skin is hot.
   B. skin is cool.

4. ____ **A.** pupils are widely dilated.
   B. pupils are constricted.

5. ____ **A.** victim feels hungry.
   B. victim feels nauseated.

6. ____ **A.** breathing and pulse are rapid.
   B. breathing and pulse are slow.

Check the relevant action(s).

A victim begins showing signs of shock. Which of the following would you do?

1. ____ Attempt to warm the victim.

2. ____ Give fluids to the victim.

3. ____ Handle the victim gently.

4. ____ Help a conscious victim walk around to aid blood flow to the heart.

5. ____ Place a conscious victim on his back and elevate the feet and legs, if injuries will not be aggravated.

6. ____ Elevate head of victim with head injury.

Match the position with condition/injury.

Write A, B, C, or D to show the best position for a conscious victim with each condition or injury below.

Best Position
A. On victim's side
B. Victim flat on back with legs elevated 8–12 inches
C. Semisitting and supported
D. Semisitting and inclined to the injured side

Condition or Injury

1. ____ Crushed chest injury

2. ____ Vomiting

3. ____ Unconscious

4. ____ Heart attack

5. ____ Head injury

6. ____ Stroke

7. ____ Amputated fingers

■ ACTIVITY 2 ■
Fainting

Mark each statement true (T) or false (F).

1. ____ Lack of oxygen to the brain causes fainting.

2. ____ Recovery within 5 minutes usually occurs after a fainting episode.

3. ____ A person may report feeling dizzy or seeing spots just before fainting.

4. ____ When a person's face becomes red and dry, fainting may occur.

Mark each action yes (Y) or no (N).

What should you do for a person turning pale and saying he feels dizzy?

1. ____ Prevent him from falling.

2. ____ Place a cold towel on his forehead.

3. ____ Loosen clothing around the person's neck.

4. ____ Place him in a semisitting position.

Choose the best answer.

What should you do for a person who suddenly collapses and falls to the floor?

1. ____ A. Pour water on his face.
   B. Wipe his face with a cool, wet cloth.

2. ____ A. Loosen clothing around victim's neck.
   B. Do not bother about loosening clothing.

3. ____ A. Elevate feet and legs.
   B. Place victim in a semisitting position.

4. ____ A. Use smelling salts or ammonia inhalants.
   B. Do *not* use smelling salts or ammonia inhalants.

5. ____ A. Seek medical help if victim does not recover within 5 minutes.
   B. Seek medical help for all fainting episodes.

■ ACTIVITY 3 ■
Anaphylactic Shock

Check the causes of anaphylactic (allergic reaction) shock in sensitive people.

1. ____ Sting by honeybee

2. ____ Eating nuts

3. ____ Taking penicillin

Check the signs and symptoms of anaphylactic shock.

1. ____ Blueness around lips and mouth

2. ____ Coughing and/or wheezing

3. ____ Breathing difficulty

4. ____ Severe itching or hives

5. ____ Nausea and vomiting

6. ____ Bleeding from the nose

7. ____ Extreme thirst

Mark each statement true (T) or false (F) regarding anaphylactic shock.

1. ____ Though the victim appears in distress, these reactions are *not* life-threatening.

2. ____ The only really effective treatment for severe allergic reaction is an immediate injection of epinephrine.

3. ____ Antihistamines are effective alone.

4. ____ Epinephrine is only available through a physician's prescription.

5. ____ Some cases require CPR.

6. ____ Several doses of epinephrine may be needed.

5

Bleeding and Wounds

■ External Bleeding ■ Internal Bleeding ■ Wounds ■
■ Tetanus ■ Amputations ■ Animal Bites ■

The average-sized adult has about six quarts of blood and can safely lose a pint during a blood donation. However, rapid blood loss of one quart or more can lead to shock and death. A child losing one pint is in extreme danger.

Blood can be lost from arteries, veins, or capillaries. Most bleeding involves more than one type of blood vessel. Blood from arteries is bright red and spurts. Arterial bleeding produces the fastest blood loss, is the most difficult to control, and is therefore the most dangerous.

Blood from a vein flows steadily and appears to be darker red. Blood oozes slowly from capillaries. Though each blood vessel contains blood differing in shades of red, an inexperienced person may have difficulty detecting the difference. The two basic types of bleeding are external and internal.

External Bleeding

This type involves visible blood coming from a wound. In most cases, bleeding stops after 5 to 10 minutes with proper first aid.

First Aid

Several methods can control or stop bleeding. They appear below in the order to be tried:

1. *Direct pressure.* Most external bleeding can be controlled by direct pressure over the wound. Steps in applying direct pressure:
   a. Place a sterile gauze dressing directly over the wound and press against it. If a sterile gauze dressing is not available, use a handkerchief, towel, or any available clean cloth.
   b. If possible, wear latex or vinyl gloves, or use other methods (e.g., extra layers of gauze, plastic wrap) for protection from the victim's blood. Afterwards, wash your hands with soap and water. When gauze dressings, latex gloves, or other protective barriers are not available and speed is important, put your bare hand and/or fingers on the wound and press to stop the blood flow.
   c. Apply a pressure bandage over the gauze dressing and wound to free yourself to perform other first aid. The dressing is best held in place with a roller bandage wrapped tightly over the dressing and above and below the wound site.
   d. Do *not* remove a dressing once it is in place because bleeding may start again. If a dressing becomes blood-soaked, apply another dressing on top of the blood-soaked one and hold them both in place.
   e. If bleeding does not stop, apply more pressure.
   f. After bleeding has stopped, maintain pressure with a bandage.

2. *Elevation.* If bleeding persists, continue applying direct pressure and elevate the extremity above the heart level. Elevation alone will not stop bleeding. Gravity helps reduce blood pressure and thus slows bleeding to allow clotting. Do *not* elevate a broken extremity.

3. *Pressure points.* If bleeding still continues, apply pressure at a pressure point while still applying direct pressure. A wound may be supplied by more than one major blood vessel, so using the pressure point alone is rarely enough to control severe bleeding.

A pressure point exists where an artery is near the skin's surface, and where it passes close to a bone against which it can be compressed. Two locations on both sides of the body are usually used to control most external bleeding cases. These are the brachial point in the arm and the femoral point in the groin.

Using pressure points requires a skillful first aider. Unless the exact location of the pulse point is known, the pressure point technique is useless.

4. *Tourniquet.* Tourniquets are rarely, if ever, necessary. Use a tourniquet only as a last resort to save a life when all other methods have failed. If used, there is a great chance of losing an arm or leg. If used, apply wide, flat materials—never rope or wire, and do *not* loosen it.

■ BLEEDING ■

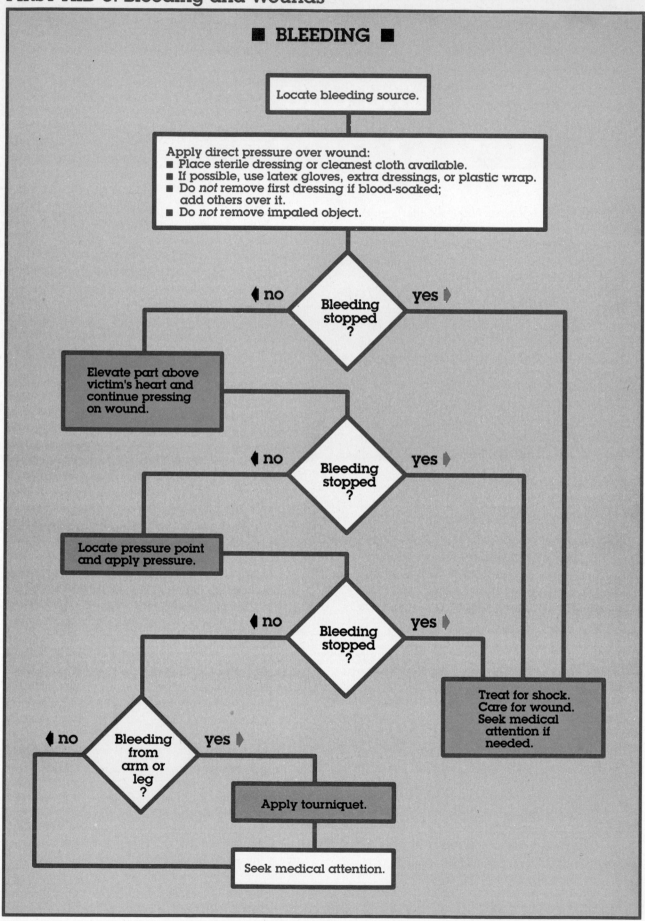

Locate bleeding source.

Apply direct pressure over wound:
- Place sterile dressing or cleanest cloth available.
- If possible, use latex gloves, extra dressings, or plastic wrap.
- Do *not* remove first dressing if blood-soaked; add others over it.
- Do *not* remove impaled object.

Bleeding stopped?

no / yes

Elevate part above victim's heart and continue pressing on wound.

Bleeding stopped?

no / yes

Locate pressure point and apply pressure.

Bleeding stopped?

no / yes

Treat for shock. Care for wound. Seek medical attention if needed.

Bleeding from arm or leg?

no / yes

Apply tourniquet.

Seek medical attention.

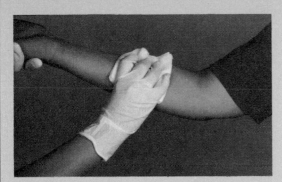

1.

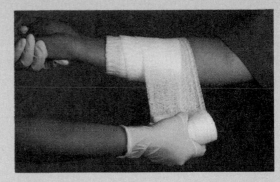

2.

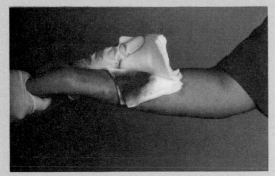

3.

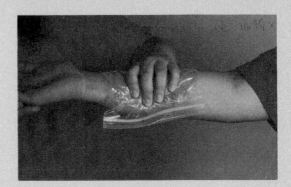

4.

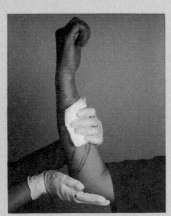

5.

1. Direct pressure stops most bleeding. Place sterile gauze pad or clean cloth over wound. Wear disposable gloves. If bleeding does not stop in 10 minutes, press harder over a wider area.

2. A pressure bandage can free you to attend to other injuries or victims.

3. Do not remove a blood-soaked dressing. Add more on top.

4. If disposable gloves are not available, use another barrier or extra gauze pads or cloths.

5. If bleeding persists, use elevation to help reduce blood flow. It must be combined with direct pressure over the wound.

6. If bleeding still continues, apply pressure at a pressure point to slow blood flow. Locations are: (A) brachial or (B) femoral. Use with direct pressure over the wound.

Tourniquets are rarely needed.

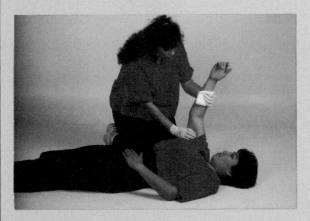

6A. Brachial

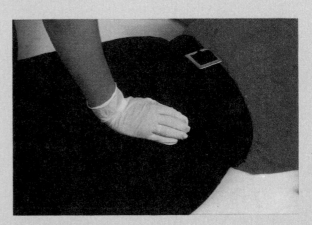

6B. Femoral

Bloodborne pathogens are disease-causing microorganisms that may be present in human blood. Two significant pathogens are Hepatitis B Virus (HBV) and Human Immunodeficiency Virus (HIV). A number of bloodborne diseases other than HIV and HBV exist, such as Hepatitis C, Hepatitis D, and syphilis.

The HBV attacks the liver. HBV is very infectious and can cause:

- Active hepatitis B—a flu-like illness that can last for months.
- A chronic carrier state—the person may have no symptoms, but can pass HBV to others
- Cirrhosis, liver cancer, and death

Fortunately, vaccines are available to prevent HBV infection. Even if you are vaccinated against HBV, you must follow the "universal precautions"—treating all blood and certain human body fluids as if they are known to be infected with bloodborne pathogens.

HIV causes AIDS (Acquired Immune Deficiency Syndrome). HIV attacks the immune system, making the body less able to fight off infections. In most cases, these infections eventually prove fatal. At present there is no vaccine to prevent infection and no known cure for AIDS.

Use personal protective equipment whenever possible while giving first aid:

1. Keep open wounds covered with dressings to prevent contact with blood.

2. Use latex gloves in every situation involving blood or other body fluids.

3. If latex gloves are not available, use the most waterproof material available or extra gauze dressings to form a barrier.

4. Whenever possible, use a mouth-to-barrier device for protection when doing rescue breathing. There may be blood in the mouth (see Appendix C).

After a person is exposed to blood or other body fluids:

1. Wash the exposed area immediately with soap and running water. Scrub vigorously with lots of lather.

2. Report the incident promptly, according to your workplace policy.

3. Get medical help, treatment, and counseling. If your workplace is covered by OSHA's Bloodborne Standards, your employer must keep medical records confidential.

4. Ask about HBV globulin (HBIG) if you haven't had the HBV vaccine. It can provide short-term protection. It's followed by vaccination against HBV.

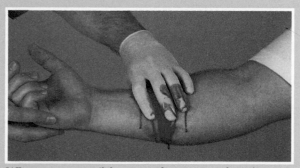

Whenever possible, use gloves as a barrier.

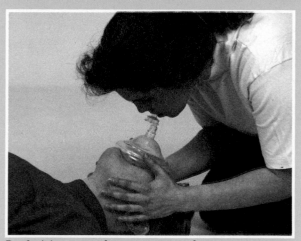

Pocket face mask, one-way valve

Internal Bleeding

Internal bleeding occurs when the skin is unbroken, and is not usually visible.

Signs and Symptoms

- Blood from the mouth (vomit, sputum) or rectum, or blood in the urine
- Nonmenstrual bleeding from the vagina
- Bruise or contusion
- Rapid pulse
- Cold and moist skin
- Dilated pupils
- Nausea and vomiting
- Painful, tender, rigid, bruised abdomen
- Fractured ribs or bruises on chest

First Aid

For severe internal bleeding:

- Monitor breathing and pulse.
- Expect vomiting. Do *not* give any liquids. If vomiting occurs, keep the victim lying on his or her side for drainage.

- Treat for shock by raising the victim's legs 8–12 inches and keeping the victim warm.
- Seek immediate medical attention.

For bruises:

- Apply an ice pack. Protect the victim's skin from frostbite by having a cloth between the ice and the skin.
- Elevate the injured part if it is not broken.
- If an arm or leg is involved, apply an elastic bandage. Do *not* apply it too tightly.

Wounds

Wounds are divided into two types: closed or open. An open wound has a break in the skin's surface with visible bleeding. A closed wound involves damage beneath the skin's surface. The skin remains unbroken, and no blood is seen.

Open Wounds

These types of wounds have damaged skin, involve visible bleeding, and could become infected.

Types of Open Wounds

- *Abrasion.* Scraped skin resulting in partial loss of the skin surface. It has little bleeding but can be very painful and serious if it covers a large area or if foreign matter becomes embedded in it.

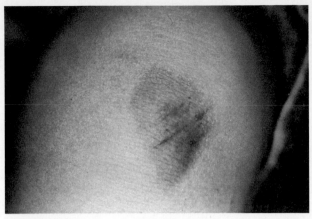

Abrasion

- *Incision.* The wound is smooth-edged and bleeds freely. The amount of bleeding depends upon the depth, location, and size of the wound. There may be severe damage to muscles, nerves, and tendons if the wound is deep.
- *Laceration.* A skin cut with jagged, irregular edges. It can bleed freely.
- *Puncture.* This is a stab from a pointed object. The entrance wound is usually small. Special treatment of the puncture wound may be required when the object causing the injury remains impaled in the wound.
- *Avulsion.* This is the tearing of a patch of skin or other tissue that is not totally torn from the body and leaves a loose, hanging

TABLE 5-1 Types of Open Wounds

Type	Cause(s)	Signs and Symptoms	First Aid
Abrasion (scrape)	Rubbing or scraping	Only skin surface affected	Remove all debris.
		Little bleeding	Wash away from wound with soap and water.
Incision (cut)	Sharp objects	Smooth edges of wound	Control bleeding.
		Severe bleeding	Wash wound.
Laceration (tearing)	Blunt object tearing skin	Veins and arteries can be affected	Control bleeding.
		Severe bleeding	Wash wound.
		Danger of infection	
Puncture (stab)	Sharp pointed object piercing skin	Wound is narrow and deep into veins and arteries	Do not remove impaled objects.
		Embedded objects	
		Danger of infection	
Avulsion (torn off)	Machinery, Explosives	Tissue torn off or left hanging	Control bleeding.
		Severe bleeding	Take avulsed part to medical facility.

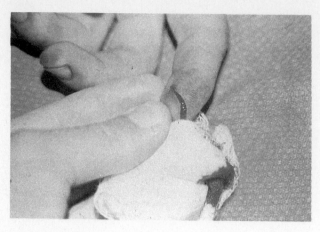

Laceration

flap. Avulsions can involve such parts as ears, fingers, hands, and even eyeballs.

- **Amputation.** This involves the cutting or tearing off of a body part such as fingers, toes, hands, feet, arms, or legs. See page 57 for more information.

First Aid

- Remove any clothing covering the wound.
- Protect against exposure to AIDS or hepatitis by wearing latex gloves or using other methods of protection (e.g., extra layers of dressings, plastic material).
- Control bleeding by applying pressure while using a dry sterile dressing or clean cloth over the entire wound. Refer to the proper steps above and under the topic of bleeding.
- Do *not* remove an impaled (penetrating) object.
- Save amputated part(s).

Cleaning wounds

For minor wounds (not seen by a physician):
- Wash your hands in a vigorous scrubbing action, using soap and water.
- Using a sterile gauze pad or a clean cloth saturated with soap and water, gently wash away from the wound edges. Foreign bodies (e.g., dirt, gravel) should be removed to avoid infection and a tattoo look after the skin heals.
- Flush the wound with large amounts of water and dry it with a sterile gauze.
- Rubbing alcohol might be used as an antiseptic on the intact skin around the wound, *not* in the wound.
- Do not put mercurochrome, merthiolate, or iodine on a wound. They kill few bacteria, can damage the skin, and many people are allergic to them.

- Cover the wound with a sterile gauze dressing and bandage. Dressings are most needed during the first 24 hours after an injury. A "band-aid" type of dressing is useful on small cuts. The dressing should *not* be airtight because it might trap moisture given off by the skin, which would encourage bacteria growth. One of the "nonstickable" dressings works well for abrasions.
- Dressings and bandages are two different kinds of first aid supplies. *Dressings* are applied over the wound to control bleeding and prevent contamination. *Bandages* hold the dressings in place. A dressing should be sterile or as clean as possible; bandages need not be.
- A skin-wound ointment with antibiotics appeals to many people. If used, apply a small amount over the wound and cover with a sterile dressing. The antibiotic can be applied several times daily. Many skin-wound protectants containing antibiotics are available. If stitches may be needed do *not* apply ointment.
- If a wound bleeds after a dressing is applied and the dressing becomes stuck, leave it on as long as the wound is healing. Pulling the scab loose to change the dressing retards healing and increases the chance of infection. If a dressing must be removed, soak it in warm water or hydrogen peroxide to help soften the scab and make removal easier.
- If a dressing becomes wet, change it. A wet dressing provides an excellent place for bacteria. Dirty dressings should be changed for a better appearance.

For severe wounds, to be seen by a physician the first aider should:
- Protect against AIDS and hepatitis by wearing latex or vinyl gloves or using a plastic wrap or extra amounts of gauze dressings.
- Remove clothing covering the wound.
- Control bleeding as described previously.
- Prevent contamination by applying a dry, sterile dressing. Do *not* wash the wound. Leave wound cleaning to a physician. If in a remote situation with medical care many hours away, clean the wound if possible, making certain that bleeding is controlled.

Closed Wounds

A bruise (contusion) results when a blunt object strikes the body. The skin is not broken and no blood appears on the skin's surface.

Signs and symptoms include: discoloration, swelling, pain, redness, and loss of use.

First Aid

- Control bleeding by applying ice and an elastic bandage immediately to the injury. Cold constricts blood vessels and thus slows bleeding. Compression over the area also helps decrease bleeding.
- Suspect and check for a fracture.
- Elevate the injured part above the victim's heart level to decrease swelling and pain.

Wounds Requiring Medical Attention

Everyone will have to make a decision about obtaining medical assistance for a wounded victim. To help in this decision, look for the following signs:

- Arterial bleeding
- Uncontrolled bleeding
- Deep incisions, lacerations, or avulsions that:
    1. Go into the muscle or bone
    2. Are located on a body part that bends (e.g., elbows or knees)
    3. Tend to gape widely
    4. Are located on the thumb or palm of hand (because nerves may be affected)
- Large and deep punctures
- Large embedded objects or deeply embedded objects of any size
- Foreign matter left in wound
- Human and animal bites
- Wounds where a scar would be noticeable. Stitched cuts usually heal with less scarring than unstitched ones.
- Eyelid cuts (to prevent later drooping)
- Slit lips (easily scarred)
- Internal bleeding
- Any wound that a first aider is *not* certain how to treat

Stitches

If stitches are needed they should be made by a physician within six to eight hours of the injury. Stitching wounds allows faster healing, reduces infection, and reduces scarring.

Wounds *not* usually requiring stitches include:

1. Those in which the skin's cut edges tend to fall together
2. Cuts less than one inch long that are not deep

Gaping wounds may be closed by using a "butterfly" bandage if all of the following are found:

1. The wound is less than eight hours old;

2. The wound is very clean; and

3. It is impossible to get to a physician because of distance.

Tetanus

Tetanus is caused by a toxin produced by a bacterium. The bacterium forms a spore that can survive in a variety of environments for years. It has been found in soil and air samples throughout the world, on human skin, and in human and animal feces.

The bacterium by itself does not cause tetanus. But when it enters a wound that contains little oxygen (e.g., a puncture wound), it can produce a toxin, which is a powerful poison. The toxin travels through the nervous system to the brain and spinal cord. It then causes contractions of certain muscle groups (particularly in the jaw). There is no known antidote to the toxin once it enters the nervous system.

The World Health Organization reports 50,000 deaths each year from tetanus, but some authorities estimate that the disease may kill as many as one million people each year. Because of good medical care in the United States, about 100 deaths a year are reported.

Vaccination can completely prevent the disease. Everyone needs a series of vaccinations to prepare the immune system to defend against the toxin. Then a booster shot once every 10 years is sufficient to jog the immune system's memory.

People who are wounded a long time after their last vaccination (e.g., 10 years) or those who did not receive all the recommended vaccinations early in life may not be able to defend themselves adequately against the tetanus toxin. In such cases, physicians can administer solutions of tetanus antibodies.

Amputations

An amputation can be one of the more gruesome wounds seen.

Types of Amputations

Amputations can be classified according to the type of injury (crushing or guillotine) and the extent of injury (partial or complete). A crushing amputation, which is the more common type, has a poor chance of reattachment. A guillotine-type of amputation has a much better chance because it is clean-cut. Microsurgical techniques can allow amputated parts to sometimes be replaced so they function normally or nearly normally.

A complete amputation may not involve heavy blood loss. This is because blood vessels tend to go into a spasm, recede into the injured body parts, and shrink in diameter, resulting in a surprisingly small blood loss. More blood is seen in a partial amputation.

First Aid

- Apply direct pressure to the bleeding site and elevate any involved extremity. Pressure on the supplying main artery (brachial or femoral) can also help in cases of severe bleeding. Tourniquets are rarely needed or used.
- Recover the amputated body part. It is best to take the amputated part to the hospital with the victim. However, in multicasualty cases, in reduced lighting conditions, or when untrained people transport the victim, someone may be requested to locate and take the missing body part to the hospital after the victim's departure. If possible, use clean water to rinse off debris—do *not* scrub.

  Studies indicate that amputated body parts without oxygen or cooling for more than six hours without cooling have little chance of survival; 24 hours is probably the maximum time allowable for an adequately cooled part.
- Care for the amputated body part by following these procedures:

  1. Rinse the part with clean water to remove any contamination—do *not* scrub.

  2. Wrap the amputated part with a dry sterile gauze or other available dry, clean cloth. Do *not* submerge the wrapped body part in water or ice. The use of a wet or moist wrapping next to the skin and tissue of an amputated part is controversial. Since either can cause water logging and tissue softening, thus affecting the chances of being successfully reattached, do *not* wrap in a moistened or damp material.

  3. If a plastic bag or waterproof container (e.g., cup or glass) is available, put the wrapped amputated part in it.

  4. Place the bag or container with the wrapped amputated part on a bed of ice, but do *not* bury it. Reattaching frostbitten parts is usually unsuccessful.

  5. Transport the part immediately to the hospital.
- If the injured part is still partially attached to the stump by a tendon or small skin "bridge," the first aid is essentially the same. Control bleeding. Wrap the part in a dry sterile dressing and place a cold pack on it. The part can still be wrapped and ice can be placed on it after it is repositioned in the normal position. Do *not* cut the "bridge" attaching the injured part.

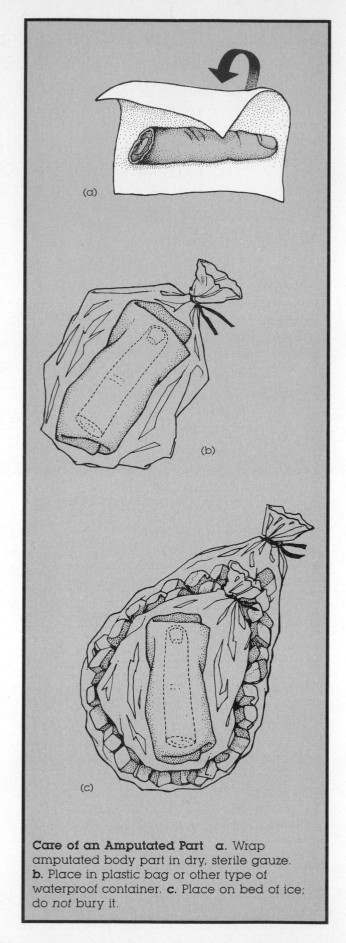

Care of an Amputated Part a. Wrap amputated body part in dry, sterile gauze. **b.** Place in plastic bag or other type of waterproof container. **c.** Place on bed of ice; do *not* bury it.

■ AMPUTATION ■

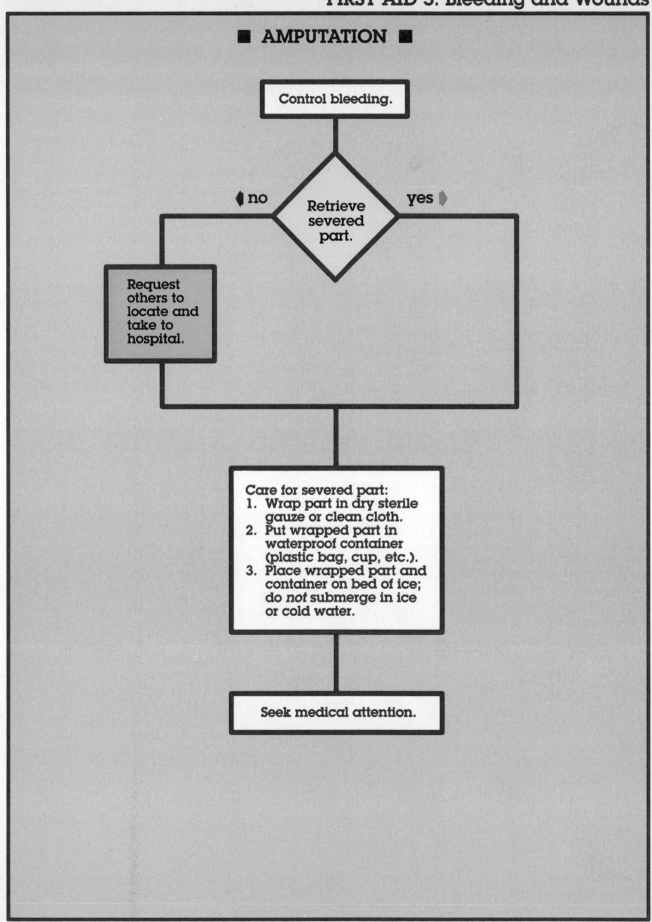

Control bleeding.

Retrieve severed part.

no → Request others to locate and take to hospital.

yes

Care for severed part:
1. Wrap part in dry sterile gauze or clean cloth.
2. Put wrapped part in waterproof container (plastic bag, cup, etc.).
3. Place wrapped part and container on bed of ice; do *not* submerge in ice or cold water.

Seek medical attention.

Animal Bites

Animal bites rarely cause lethal bleeding, but they can produce significant damage. Sixty to 90% of the animal bites in the United States come from dogs. The annual number of dog bites has been estimated to be between one to two million cases.

Animal bites of all kinds account for about one percent of all hospital emergency department visits. About one bite in 10 needs stitches, but all bites require complete cleaning, which may be impossible by a first aider.

A dog's mouth may carry more than 60 different species of bacteria, some of which are very dangerous to humans (e.g., rabies). Human, cat, and other animal bites are equally contaminated and dangerous.

First Aid

- If the wound is not bleeding heavily, wash it with soap and water. Washing should take five to 10 minutes. Scrubbing can traumatize tissues, so avoid it whenever possible. Allowing a wound to bleed a little helps remove bacteria left in the tissues.
- Rinse the wound thoroughly with running water.
- Control bleeding with direct pressure, and if an extremity is involved and the bleeding continues, use elevation along with the direct pressure.
- Cover with a sterile dressing, but do *not* seal the wound tightly with tape or butterfly bandages.
- Seek medical attention because of the danger of infection, need for further cleaning, the possible need for a tetanus shot and stitches to close the wound.

Rabies

Although many people are still concerned about the possibility of getting rabies from dogs, 96% of the rabies cases seen in the United States come from skunks, raccoons, and bats. During a recent year, about 100 rabid dogs were reported nationally, and those dogs did not always bite someone.

Only one or two cases of human rabies occur in the United States each year, and they generally originate outside the country. Since there is no cure for rabies, few victims survive it. In fact, only two cases of survival have been reported in medical history. A virus found in warm-blooded animals causes rabies and spreads from one animal to another, usually through a bite or by licking involving saliva from an infected animal.

Bites from animals that are not warm-blooded (e.g., snakes, reptiles) do not carry the danger of rabies. However, such bites can become infected and should be washed well and watched for signs of infection.

Avoiding Dog Bites

With an estimated 1 to 2 million Americans bitten by dogs each year, everyone should attempt to avoid being bitten. The U.S. postal system offers advice about dogs to its carriers which could be of use to others:

1. **Observe the area.** Take a quick glance at all places a dog could be—under parked cars or hedges, on the porch, etc.

2. **Size up the situation.** Is the dog asleep, barking, growling, nonchalant, large, small, etc?

3. **Avoid showing signs of fear.** A dog is more apt to bite if he knows you are afraid of him.

4. **Don't startle a dog.** If he is asleep, make some kind of nonstartling noise, such as a whistle. Do this before you are close to him, while you still have time for an "out."

5. **Never assume a dog won't bite.** You may encounter a certain dog for days or weeks without incident, but one day he may decide to bite you.

6. **Keep your eyes on the dog.** A dog is basically a coward and a sneak, and is more likely to bite you when you aren't looking.

7. **Make friends.** Talk in a friendly tone of voice, call his name if you know it, but don't attempt to pet him.

8. **Stand your ground.** If a dog comes toward you, turn and face him; if you have a satchel, hold it in front of you and back slowly away, making sure you don't stumble and fall. By all means, never turn and run.

9. **Never walk between a dog and its master,** and never walk toward children when a dog is present, because it may take action to defend them.

What to Do in Case of a Bite

- Try to locate the animal's owner or in the case of a wild animal find its location. Call the EMS, police, or animal control to capture it. Do *not* try to capture the animal yourself, and keep away from it. The health department will observe the captured animal for possible rabies. When the animal cannot be found or identified, the bitten victim must usually go through a series of rabies shots (vaccination).
- Do *not* kill the animal. If it is killed, protect the head and brain from damage so they can be examined for rabies. If it is dead, transport the animal intact to prevent exposure to the potentially infected tissues or saliva. If necessary, the animal's remains can be refrigerated (avoid freezing).
- Give first aid as described above and seek medical attention for a possible series of vaccine inoculations and stitches to close the wound.

Human Bites

Human bites can cause a very severe injury—more often than animal bites do. The human mouth contains a wide range of bacteria and the likelihood of infection is greater from a human bite than from other warm-blooded animals.

Types of Human Bites

There are two kinds of human bites:

1. *True bites.* These occur when any part of the body's flesh is caught between teeth. These bites happen during fights between children and between adults and in cases involving abuse of children, spouses, and elders.

2. *Fight bites.* These occur when the victim cuts his or her knuckles on another person's teeth. Though these injuries usually result from a deliberate action (e.g., during a fight), unintentional injury can happen during sports and play (e.g., basketball).

First Aid

First aid involves:

- Thoroughly washing the wound with soap and water
- Applying a dry, sterile dressing and seeking medical attention

■ ANIMAL BITES ■

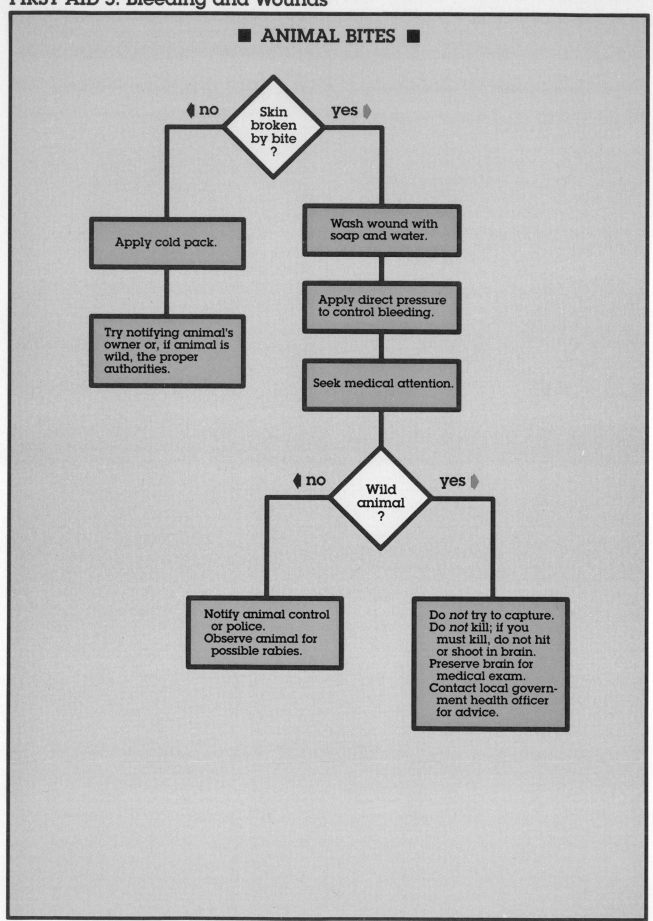

Skin broken by bite?

← **no**

yes →

Apply cold pack.

Try notifying animal's owner or, if animal is wild, the proper authorities.

Wash wound with soap and water.

Apply direct pressure to control bleeding.

Seek medical attention.

Wild animal?

← **no**

yes →

Notify animal control or police.
Observe animal for possible rabies.

Do *not* try to capture.
Do *not* kill; if you must kill, do not hit or shoot in brain.
Preserve brain for medical exam.
Contact local government health officer for advice.

■ ACTIVITY 1 ■
External Bleeding and Wounds

Mark each statement true (T) or false (F).

1. _____ Loss of blood occurs only in open wounds.
2. _____ A bruise on the thigh is an example of an external wound.
3. _____ Closed wounds occur when blood vessels beneath the skin have been broken.
4. _____ Bleeding from veins is usually fast and in spurts.
5. _____ Losing more than a quart of blood for an adult is life-threatening.
6. _____ Completely severed arteries bleed more freely than partially cut arteries.
7. _____ Arterial bleeding is usually more serious than venous bleeding.

Check (✓) the appropriate action(s).

Which of the following actions should be taken to control bleeding when blood is flowing freely from a wound?

1. _____ Press tightly on the wound.
2. _____ If arm is elevated to control bleeding, stop direct pressure.
3. _____ Use a femoral pressure point alone if direct pressure fails to stop the bleeding.

Mark each statement true (T) or false (F).

1. _____ When washing a wound with soap and water, wash toward the wound.
2. _____ Hydrogen peroxide kills bacteria (germs) in a wound.
3. _____ If using rubbing alcohol, apply it on the skin around the wound, not in the wound.
4. _____ A butterfly bandage can be used to bring small cut skin edges together.
5. _____ If a dressing must be removed and part of the scab sticks to it, soak the dressing in warm water for easier removal.
6. _____ Cuts to eyelids and lips should be stitched by a physician.
7. _____ Stitches can be placed by a physician hours after the injury occurred.

Choose the best answer regarding types of wounds.

1. _____ A smooth cut made by a sharp object, such as a razor blade, is called:
   A. An incision
   B. A laceration
   C. An avulsion
   D. An abrasion
2. _____ Skinned elbows and knees are examples of:
   A. Hematomas
   B. Avulsions
   C. Lacerations
   D. Abrasions
3. _____ Which type of wound has a jagged cut where the tissues are snagged and torn, forming a rough edge around the wound?
   A. Incision
   B. Laceration
   C. Contusion
   D. Hematoma
4. _____ The most common form of closed wound is:
   A. Abrasion
   B. Contusion
   C. Laceration
   D. Incision
5. _____ Which type of wound is caused by sharp, pointed objects such as nails, splinters, or knives?
   A. Abrasion
   B. Avulsion
   C. Puncture
   D. Contusion
6. _____ Which of the following is most susceptible to tetanus?
   A. Laceration
   B. Amputation
   C. Incision
   D. Puncture
7. _____ Which of the following describes bleeding from a vein?
   A. Bright red, flowing steadily
   B. Bright red, spurting
   C. Dark maroon, flowing steadily
   D. Dark maroon, spurting

Choose the best answer regarding dressings.

1. _____ The material used to hold sterile material over a wound:
   A. Must be sterile
   B. Must be adhesive
   C. Is a dressing
   D. Is a bandage

2. _____ Any material applied directly to a wound in an effort to control bleeding and prevent further contamination:
   A. Is a bandage
   B. Is a dressing
   C. Should not be sterile
   D. Should be loosely secured to help in checking the wound

3. _____ Use of a sterile dressing on an open wound will:
   A. Reduce further contamination
   B. Kill any bacteria present in the wound
   C. Only be necessary if the wound is bleeding profusely
   D. Prevent shock

4. _____ After a dressing has been applied to a wound, if bleeding continues, the first aider should:
   A. Remove the blood-soaked dressing and replace it with a clean, sterile dressing
   B. Leave the original dressing in place and place a new dressing over the blood-soaked ones

■ ACTIVITY 2 ■
Infection and Tetanus

Prevent infection by:

1. _____ Immediately washing a wound with soap and water

2. _____ Getting a tetanus booster shot every year

3. _____ Applying rubbing or ethyl alcohol directly on the wound

4. _____ Using mercurochrome or merthiolate instead of soap and water

5. _____ Using any one of several recommended skin-wound protectants

■ ACTIVITY 3 ■
Amputation

Mark each statement true (T) or false (F).

1. _____ Usually small blood loss occurs in complete amputation.

2. _____ An amputated part has little chance of survival.

3. _____ Bury an amputated part in ice.

4. _____ Cut off a partially attached part.

5. _____ Locate any amputated part, regardless of size, and take it to the nearest medical facility.

6. _____ Amputated parts older than six hours without proper cooling have little chance of survival.

7. _____ Wrap the amputated part with a wet or moist dressing.

■ ACTIVITY 4 ■
Animal Bites

Mark each statement true (T) or false (F).

1. _____ Most dog bites should be treated by a physician.

2. _____ In most cases, wash the wound with soap and water before attempting to stop bleeding.

3. _____ Washing the wound should take only one or two minutes.

4. _____ Control bleeding with direct pressure.

5. _____ Human and cat bites are not as dangerous as dog bites.

6. _____ Kill the biting animal so the brain can be inspected for rabies.

7. _____ Pet animals are the leading rabies carriers.

8. _____ Both warm- and cold-blooded animals carry rabies.

6

Specific Body Area Injuries

■ Head Injuries ■ Eye Injuries ■ Nosebleeds ■ Dental Injuries ■ Chest Injuries ■
■ Abdominal Injuries ■ Finger and Toe Injuries ■ Fishhook Removal ■
■ Ring Removal ■ Blisters ■

Head Injuries

Scalp Wounds

Scalp wounds bleed profusely because of the scalp's rich blood supply. Look in the wound for skull bone or brain exposure and indentation of the skull.

- Control bleeding by gently applying direct pressure with a dry sterile dressing. If it becomes blood-filled, do *not* remove it but add another dressing on top of the first one.
- If a depressed skull fracture is suspected, apply pressure around the edges of the wound rather than at its center.
- Elevate the head and shoulders to help control bleeding.
- Do *not* remove an impaled object; instead, immobilize it in place with bulky dressings.

Skull Fracture

A skull fracture is a break or crack in the cranium (bony case surrounding the brain). Skull fractures may be open or closed, as with other bone fractures.

Signs and symptoms

- Pain at the point of injury
- Deformity of the skull
- Bleeding from ears and/or nose
- Leakage of clear or pink watery fluid dripping from the nose or ear. This watery fluid is known as cerebrospinal fluid (CSF). CSF can be detected by having the suspected fluid drip onto a handkerchief, pillowcase, or other cloth. CSF will form a pink ring resembling a target around the blood; this is also called the "halo sign."
- Discoloration under the eyes ("raccoon eyes")
- Discoloration behind an ear (Battle's sign)
- Unequal pupils
- Profuse scalp bleeding if skin is broken. A scalp wound may expose skull or brain tissue.

First aid for skull fractures is similar to that for a victim with a scalp wound (see above) or a brain contusion (see page 66).

Concussion

A concussion comes from a blow to the head that results in a violent jar or shaking to the brain, causing an immediate change in brain function, including possible loss of consciousness.

Signs and Symptoms

- Loss of consciousness
- Severe headache
- Memory loss (amnesia)
- Seeing stars
- Dizziness
- Weakness
- Double vision

Degrees of Concussion

Categorizing concussion helps the first aider to decide how to manage the victim. Concussions may be categorized as follows:

TABLE 6-1 Concussion Guidelines

Type	Description	Guidelines
Mild	Momentary or no loss of consciousness	Delay return to activity until medical evaluation has been made.
Moderate	Unconscious for less than five minutes	Avoid vigorous activity for a few days or longer. Resume activity only when associated symptoms of headache, visual disturbances, etc. have been resolved.
Severe	Unconscious for more than five minutes	Avoid rigorous activity for one month or longer. Clearance from a neurosurgeon is advised.

A **mild** concussion involves no loss of consciousness, but a disturbance of neurological function.

A **moderate** concussion involves a loss of consciousness for less than five minutes, usually with the inability to remember events after being injured.

In a **severe** concussion, the loss of consciousness lasts more than five minutes and eye movements wander.

Contusion

Contusions are more serious than concussions. Both can be produced by hits or blows to the head. Contusions involve bruising and swelling of the brain, with blood vessels within the brain rupturing and bleeding. Inside the skull, there is no way for the blood to escape and no room for it to accumulate.

Signs and Symptoms

- Similar to those of a concussion but more severe
- Unconsciousness
- Paralysis or weakness
- Unequal pupil size
- Vomiting and nausea
- Blurred vision
- Amnesia or memory lapses
- Headache

First Aid for Concussions and Contusions

Any head injury may be accompanied by a spinal injury. If you suspect a spinal injury, keep the head, neck, and spine in the same alignment you found originally.

For unconscious victims

- Assume that all unconscious victims of head injury have a spinal neck injury. Open the airway by the jaw thrust method to check for breathing. Do *not* bend the neck. Give rescue breathing if needed.
- Stabilize the victim's head and neck as you found them, using your hands along both sides of the head and/or placing blankets and other soft yet rigid materials alongside the head and neck.
- Check for severe bleeding. Cover any bleeding with a sterile dressing. Do *not* stop the flow of blood or fluid from the ears. Stopping it could put pressure on the brain. Do *not* remove any object embedded in the skull.
- If there are no signs of a neck or spinal injury, try to place the victim in the coma position (on victim's side, knees bent, head supported on one arm).

For conscious victims

- Check for spinal injury by noting arm or leg weakness or paralysis; if you get little or no reaction when you pinch the feet and hands, there may be a spinal injury. Stabilize the head and neck as they were found, to prevent movement.
- Do *not* block the escape of cerebrospinal fluid since it may add more pressure to the brain.
- Ask the victim what day it is, where he or she is, and personal questions such as birthday and home address. If the victim cannot answer these questions, there may be a significant

Head Injury Follow-Up

If any of the following signs appear within 48 hours of a head injury, seek medical attention:

- *Headache.* Expect a headache. If it lasts more than one or two days or increases in severity, however, seek medical advice.
- *Nausea, vomiting.* If nausea lasts more than two hours, seek medical advice. Vomiting once or twice, especially in children, may be expected after a head injury. Vomiting does not tell anything about the severity of the injury. However, if vomiting begins again hours after one or two episodes have ceased, consult a physician.
- *Drowsiness.* Allow a victim to sleep, but wake the victim at least every hour to check the state of consciousness and sense of orientation by asking his or her name, address, telephone number, and an

information-processing question (e.g., adding or multiplying numbers). If the victim cannot answer correctly or appears confused or disoriented, call a physician.
- *Vision problems.* If the victim "sees double," if the eyes fail to move together, or if one pupil appears to be larger than the other, seek medical advice.
- *Mobility.* If the victim cannot use his or her arms or legs as well as previously or is unsteady in walking, medical care should be sought.
- *Speech.* If the victim slurs his or her speech or is unable to talk, a doctor should be consulted.
- *Seizures or convulsions.* If the victim has a violent involuntary contraction (spasm) or series of contractions of the skeletal muscles, seek medical assistance.

problem. Another useful test is to give a list of five or six numbers and ask the victim to repeat them back in that order. Lists of objects can also be used as short-term memory tests. Failing on these short-term memory tests indicates a concussion.

- Keep victim in a semi-sitting position; do *not* elevate the legs since this increase blood pressure in the head.
- Do *not* give the victim anything to eat or drink.

Eye Injuries

Penetrating Injuries

Most penetrating eye injuries are fairly obvious. Suspect penetration any time you see a lid laceration or cut. Often first aiders concentrate upon the lid injury and neglect the penetrating eye injury. A penetrating injury requires immediate ophthalmological attention.

- Do *not* remove foreign bodies impaled in the eye.
- Protect the eye with padding around the object. Place a paper cup or cardboard cone to prevent the object from being driven farther into the eye.
- Cover the undamaged eye with a patch in order to stop movement of the damaged eye due to sympathetic eye movement.

Blows to the Eye*

Apply an ice cold compress immediately for about 15 minutes to reduce pain and swelling. A black eye or blurred vision could signal internal eye damage. See an ophthalmologist immediately.

Cuts of the Eye and Lid*

- Bandage both eyes lightly and seek medical help immediately.
- Do *not* attempt to wash out the eye or remove an object stuck in the eye.
- Never apply hard pressure to the injured eye or eyelid.

Chemical Injury*

- Flood the eye with warm water immediately. Use your fingers to keep the eye open as wide as possible. Hold head under a faucet or pour water into the eye from any clean container for at least 15 minutes, continuously and gently. Roll the eyeball as much as possible to

Source: American Academy of Ophthalmology; used with permission.

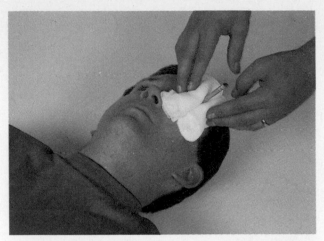

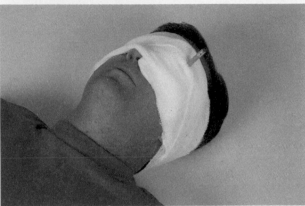

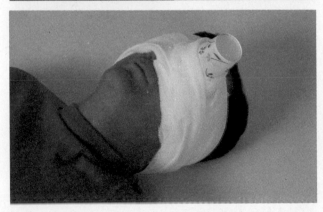

Bandaging eye (paper cup)

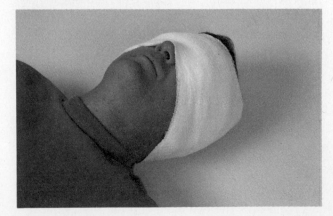

Bandaging both eyes

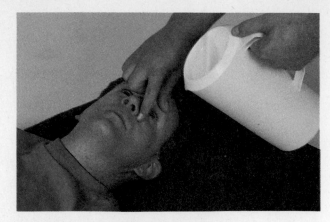

Flushing eye for chemical burn

wash out the eye. Do *not* use an eye cup.

- Loosely bandage both eyes. Seek medical help immediately after these steps are taken.

Alkalis cause greater concern than acids since they penetrate deeper and continue to damage longer. No matter how well the eye is irrigated, some alkali will always remain, often for weeks, to cause tissue damage. A first aider cannot use enough water on these injuries.

Avulsion of the Eye

A blow to the face can avulse an eye from its socket.

- Do *not* attempt to push the eye back into the socket.
- Cover the extruded eye loosely with a sterile dressing that has been moistened with clean water. Then cover the eye with a paper cup, using the same procedures for an impaled object in the eye.
- Cover the uninjured eye with a patch to prevent sympathetic eye movement in the damaged eye.

Foreign Bodies

Foreign bodies in the eye are the most frequent of eye injuries. They can be very painful. Tearing is very common, as it is the body's way of attempting to remove the object.

- Do *not* rub any speck or particle that is in the eye. Lift the upper lid over the lower lid, allowing the lashes to brush the speck off the inside of the upper lid. Blink a few times and let the eye move the particle out. If the speck remains, keep the eye closed and seek medical help.
- Try flushing the object out by rinsing the eye gently with warm water. You may have to help hold the eye open and tell the victim to move the eye as it is rinsed. If the object is on

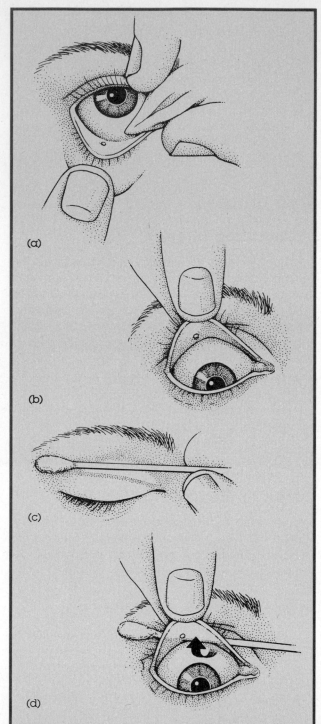

(a)

(b)

(c)

(d)

Everted Eyelid a. If tears or gentle flushing do not remove object, gently pull lower lid down. Remove an object by gently flushing with lukewarm water or a wet sterile gauze. **b.** If no object is seen inside lower lid, check the upper lid. **c.** Tell the person to look down. Pull gently downward on upper eyelashes. Lay a swab or matchstick across the top of the lid. **d.** Fold the lid over the swab or matchstick. Remove an object by gently flushing with lukewarm water or a wet sterile gauze.

■ HEAD INJURIES ■

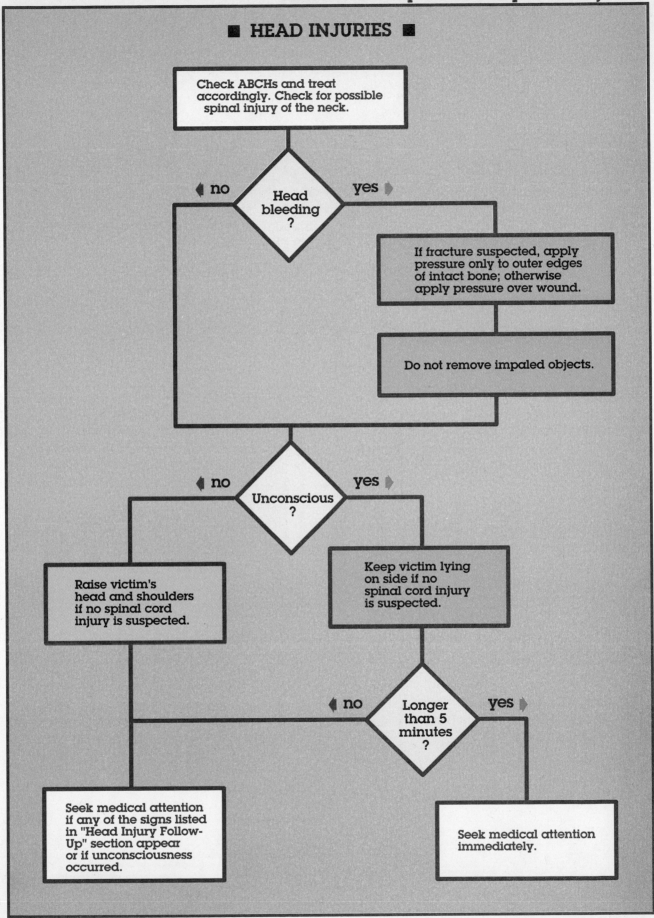

Check ABCHs and treat accordingly. Check for possible spinal injury of the neck.

Head bleeding?
no ◀ | ▶ yes

If fracture suspected, apply pressure only to outer edges of intact bone; otherwise apply pressure over wound.

Do not remove impaled objects.

Unconscious?
no ◀ | ▶ yes

Raise victim's head and shoulders if no spinal cord injury is suspected.

Keep victim lying on side if no spinal cord injury is suspected.

Longer than 5 minutes?
no ◀ | ▶ yes

Seek medical attention if any of the signs listed in "Head Injury Follow-Up" section appear or if unconsciousness occurred.

Seek medical attention immediately.

■ EYE INJURIES ■

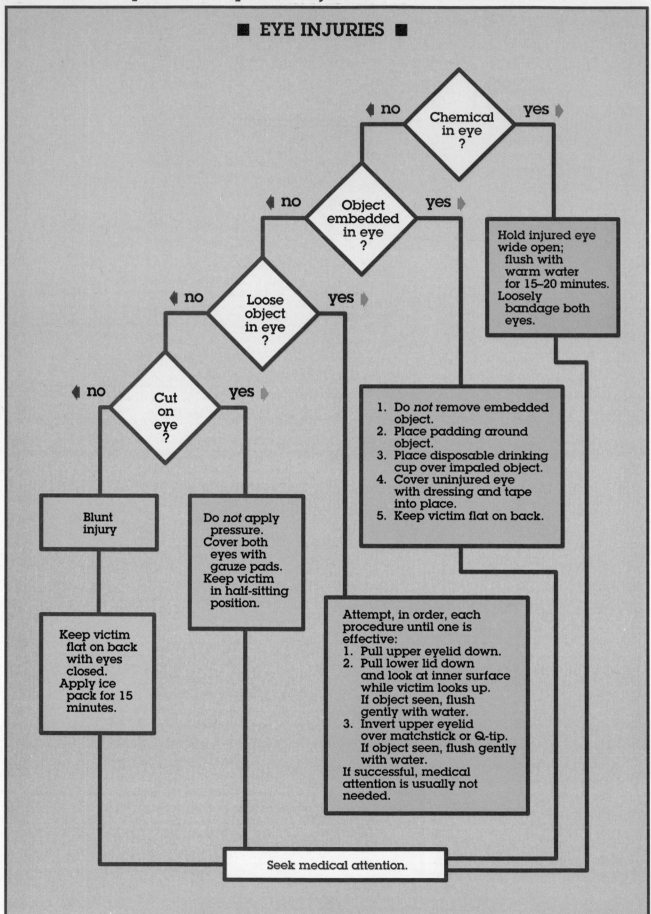

Chemical in eye ? — no / yes

Object embedded in eye ? — no / yes

Loose object in eye ? — no / yes

Cut on eye ? — no / yes

Hold injured eye wide open; flush with warm water for 15–20 minutes. Loosely bandage both eyes.

1. Do *not* remove embedded object.
2. Place padding around object.
3. Place disposable drinking cup over impaled object.
4. Cover uninjured eye with dressing and tape into place.
5. Keep victim flat on back.

Blunt injury

Do *not* apply pressure. Cover both eyes with gauze pads. Keep victim in half-sitting position.

Keep victim flat on back with eyes closed. Apply ice pack for 15 minutes.

Attempt, in order, each procedure until one is effective:
1. Pull upper eyelid down.
2. Pull lower lid down and look at inner surface while victim looks up. If object seen, flush gently with water.
3. Invert upper eyelid over matchstick or Q-tip. If object seen, flush gently with water.
If successful, medical attention is usually not needed.

Seek medical attention.

the white part of the eye, have the victim look down while rinsing the eye with water.

- If rinsing does not work, the object is probably stuck under the upper or lower lid. Examine the lower lid by pulling it down gently. If you see the object, flush the eye with water. To examine the upper lid, grasp the lashes of the upper lid, place a match stick or swab across the upper lid and roll the lid upward over the stick or swab. If you see the object, remove it with a moistened sterile gauze.

Light Burns

These injuries can result from looking at ultraviolet light (e.g., sunlight, arc welding, snowblindness). Severe pain occurs one to six hours after exposure.

- Cover both eyes with cold, moist compresses and prevent light from reaching the victim's eyes by having him or her rest in a darkened room.
- An analgesic for pain may be needed.
- Call an ophthalmologist for advice.

Contact Lenses

Determine if the victim is wearing contact lenses by asking, by checking on a driver's license, or by looking for them on the eyeball, using a light shining on the eye from the side. In cases of chemical eye burns, lenses should be immediately removed. Usually the victim can effectively remove the lenses.

Nosebleeds

Severe nosebleed frightens the victim and often challenges the first aider's skill. Most nosebleeds are self-limited and seldom require medical attention. However, in cases of accompanying head or neck injuries, stabilize the head and neck for protection. In some cases enough blood could be lost to cause shock.

Types of Nosebleeds

- *Anterior* (front of nose). The most common (90%); bleeds out of one nostril.
- *Posterior* (back of nose). Massive bleeding backward into the mouth or down the back of the throat; bleeding starts on one side, then comes out of both nostrils and down the throat; serious and requires medical attention.

First Aid

Most anterior (front of nose) nosebleeds can be stopped by these simple procedures:

- Reassure and keep the victim quiet. Though a large amount of blood may appear to have been lost, most nosebleeds are not serious.

- Keep the victim in a sitting position to reduce blood pressure.
- Keep the victim's head tilted slightly forward so that the blood can run out the front of the nose, not down the back of the throat, which causes either choking or nausea and vomiting. The vomit could be inhaled into the lungs.
- If a foreign object in the nose is suspected, look into the nose, but do *not* probe with a finger or swab.
- With thumb and forefinger, apply steady pressure to both nostrils for five minutes before releasing. Remind the victim to breathe through his or her mouth and to spit out any accumulated blood.
- If bleeding persists, have the victim gently blow the nose to remove any clots and excess blood, and to minimize sneezing. This allows new clots to form. Then, press the nostrils again for five minutes.
- Some experts recommend gently placing inside the bleeding nostril a cotton ball that has been soaked in hydrogen peroxide, a nasal decongestant, or plain water. Sometimes lack of time and/or materials prevent using this procedure.
- Some authorities suggest placing a roll of gauze (diameter of a pencil in size) between the upper lip and teeth and pressing against it with your fingers to stop the blood flow.

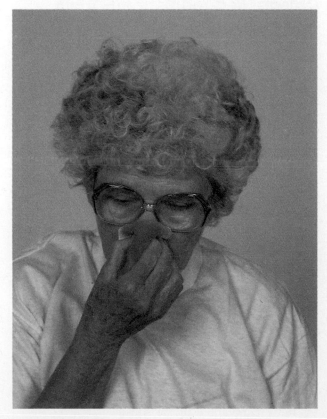

Nosebleed

- Apply ice over the nose to help control bleeding.
- If the victim is unconscious, place the victim on his or her side to prevent inhaling of blood and attempt the procedures in the above list.
- Seek medical attention if any of the following occurs:

    1. The nostril pinching does *not* stop the bleeding after a second attempt.

    2. Signs and symptoms suggest a posterior source of bleeding.

    3. The victim has high blood pressure, is taking anticoagulants (blood thinners) or large doses of aspirin.

    4. Bleeding occurs after a blow to the nose (suspect a broken nose).

Most nosebleed victims never need medical care since nosebleeds are self-limited, and the victim can control the bleeding.

Dental Injuries

The following first aid procedures provide temporary relief for dental emergencies, but it is important to consult with a dentist as soon as possible.

Objects Wedged Between Teeth

- Attempt to remove the object with dental floss. Guide the floss in carefully so the gum tissue is not injured.
- Do *not* use a sharp or pointed tool to remove the object. If unsuccessful, take the victim to a dentist.

Bitten Lip or Tongue

Apply direct pressure to the bleeding area with a sterile gauze or clean cloth. If the lip is swollen, apply a cold compress. Take the victim to a hospital emergency room if the bleeding persists or if the bite is severe.

Knocked-Out Tooth

More than 2 million teeth are accidentally knocked out in the United States each year. More than 90% of them can be saved with the proper treatment.

- When a permanent tooth is completely knocked out, save it and take it, along with the victim, to the dentist immediately. With proper first aid procedures, the tooth may be successfully reimplanted in the socket.
- Do *not* put the tooth in mouthwash or alcohol

Care After a Nosebleed

After a nosebleed has stopped, suggest to the victim:

1. Sneeze through an open mouth, if there is a need to sneeze.

2. Avoid bending over or too much physical exertion.

3. Elevate the head with two pillows when lying down.

4. Keep the nostrils moist by applying a little petroleum jelly just inside the nostril for a week; increase the humidity in the bedroom during the winter months with a cold-mist humidifier.

5. Avoid picking or rubbing the nose.

6. Avoid hot drinks and alcoholic beverages for a week.

7. Avoid smoking or taking aspirin for a week.

or scrub it with abrasives or chemicals. And do *not* touch the root of the tooth.
- Place the tooth in a cup of cold whole milk. Avoid low fat or powdered milk or milk by-products such as yogurt.
- Take the victim and tooth to a dentist immediately (within 30 minutes). Some experts recommend that the tooth be placed in the victim's mouth to keep it moist until dental treatment is available. This method, though convenient, presents the risk, especially in children, of the tooth's being accidentally swallowed.
- A partially extracted tooth can be pushed into place without rinsing the tooth. Then seek a dentist so the loose tooth can be stabilized.
- If in remote areas with no dentist nearby, replant a knocked-out tooth by first running cool water over it to clean away debris (do *not* scrub the tooth), and then by gently repositioning it in the socket, using adjacent teeth as a guide. Push the tooth so the top is even with the adjacent teeth. Successful replanting occurs best within 30 minutes of the accident. See a dentist as soon as possible.

Broken Tooth

- Immediate attention is necessary when a tooth breaks since it may need to be extracted. Attempt to clean any dirt, blood, and debris from the injured area with a sterile gauze or clean cloth and warm water.

TABLE 6-2 Dental Emergency Procedures

Toothache	Rinse the mouth vigorously with warm water to clean it out. Use dental floss to remove any food that might be trapped between the teeth. (*Do not place aspirin on the aching tooth or gum tissues.*) See the dentist as soon as possible.
Problems with braces and retainers	If a wire is causing irritation, cover the end with a small cotton ball, beeswax or a piece of gauze, until you can get to the dentist. If a wire gets stuck in the cheek, tongue or gum tissue, do not attempt to remove it. Go to the dentist immediately. If an appliance becomes loose or a piece of it breaks off, take the appliance and the piece and go to the dentist.
Knocked-out tooth	If the tooth is dirty, rinse it gently in running water. *Do not scrub it or remove any attached tissue fragments.* Gently insert and hold the tooth in its socket. If this is not possible, place the tooth in a cup of milk or a special tooth-preserving solution available at your local drugstore. If you can get to the dentist within 30 minutes, there is a good chance the tooth can be saved! Do not forget to bring the tooth!
Broken tooth	Gently clean dirt from the injured area with warm water. Place cold compresses on the face, in the area of the injured tooth, to decrease swelling. Go to the dentist immediately.
Bitten tongue or lip	Apply direct pressure to the bleeding area with a clean cloth. If swelling is present, apply cold compresses. If bleeding does not stop, go to a hospital emergency room.
Objects wedged between teeth	Try to remove the object with floss. Guide the floss carefully to avoid cutting the gums. If you're not successful in removing the object, go to the dentist. Do not try to remove the object with a sharp or pointed instrument.
Possible broken jaw	Do not move the jaw. Secure the jaw in place by tying a handkerchief, necktie or towel around the jaw and over the top of the head. If swelling is present, apply cold compresses. Go immediately to a hospital emergency room, or call the dentist.

Source: Copyright by the American Dental Association; reprinted by permission.

- Apply a cold compress on the face next to the injured tooth to minimize swelling.
- If a jaw fracture is suspected, immobilize the jaw by any available means—place a scarf, handkerchief, tie, or towel over and under the chin, and tie the ends on top of the victim's head. In either case, immediately take the victim to an oral surgeon or hospital emergency room.

- Use dental floss to remove any food that might be trapped between the teeth.
- Do *not* place aspirin on the aching tooth or gum tissues.
- If a cavity is present, insert a small cotton ball soaked in oil of cloves (eugenol). Do *not* cover a cavity with cotton if there is any pus discharge or facial swelling. See a dentist as soon as possible.

Toothache

- Rinse the mouth vigorously with warm water to clean out debris.

Although temporary relief can be provided in most dental emergencies, by all means, when in doubt, consult a dentist as soon as possible.

■ NOSEBLEEDS ■

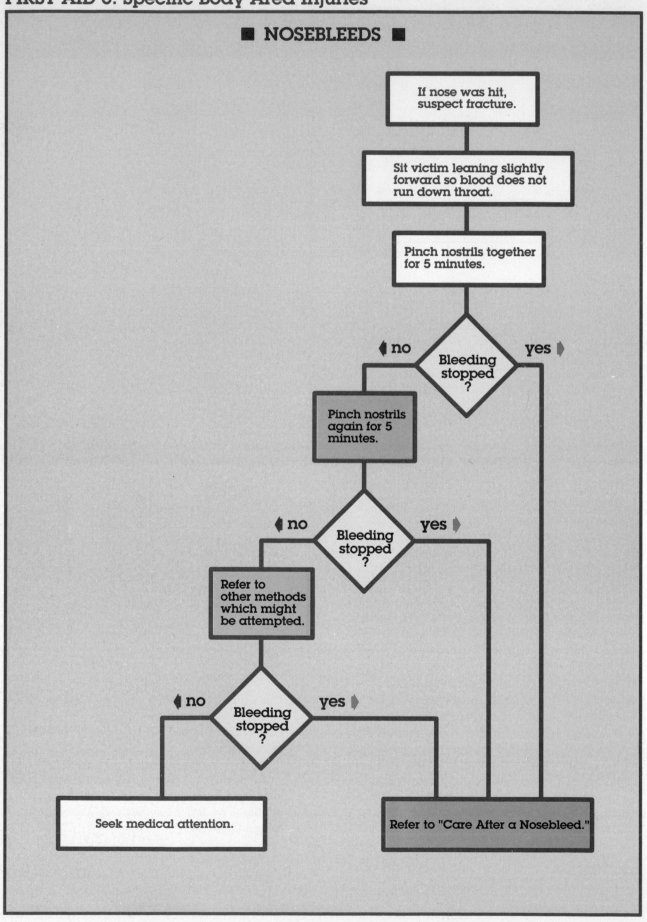

If nose was hit, suspect fracture.

Sit victim leaning slightly forward so blood does not run down throat.

Pinch nostrils together for 5 minutes.

Bleeding stopped?

◀ no   yes ▶

Pinch nostrils again for 5 minutes.

Bleeding stopped?

◀ no   yes ▶

Refer to other methods which might be attempted.

Bleeding stopped?

◀ no   yes ▶

Seek medical attention.

Refer to "Care After a Nosebleed."

■ DENTAL INJURIES ■

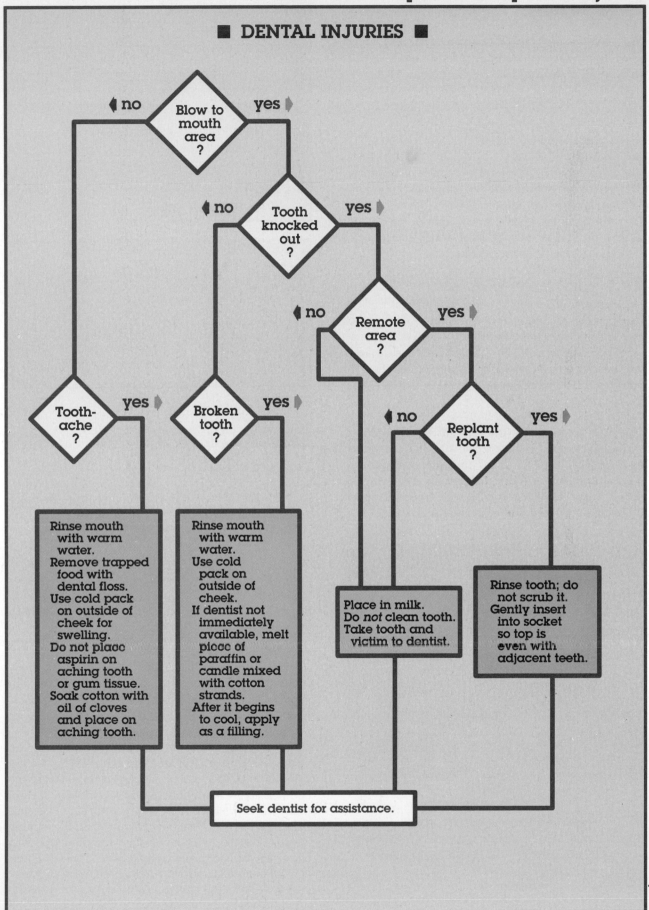

Blow to mouth area ? — no / yes

Tooth knocked out ? — no / yes

Remote area ? — no / yes

Tooth-ache ? — yes

Broken tooth ? — yes

Replant tooth ? — no / yes

Rinse mouth with warm water.
Remove trapped food with dental floss.
Use cold pack on outside of cheek for swelling.
Do not place aspirin on aching tooth or gum tissue.
Soak cotton with oil of cloves and place on aching tooth.

Rinse mouth with warm water.
Use cold pack on outside of cheek.
If dentist not immediately available, melt piece of paraffin or candle mixed with cotton strands.
After it begins to cool, apply as a filling.

Place in milk.
Do *not* clean tooth.
Take tooth and victim to dentist.

Rinse tooth; do not scrub it.
Gently insert into socket so top is even with adjacent teeth.

Seek dentist for assistance.

Chest Injuries

Chest wounds may be either **open** or **closed. Open chest wounds** are caused by penetrating objects. **Closed chest wounds** result from blunt blows.

Signs and Symptoms

Important signs of chest injuries include:

- Pain at the injury site
- Breathing difficulty
- Blueness of the lips and/or fingernail beds, indicating oxygen deficiency (cyanosis)
- Coughing or spitting up blood
- Bruising or an open chest wound
- Failure of one or both sides of the chest to expand normally when inhaling

Types of Chest Injuries and First Aid

Rib fracture. The victim can usually point out the injury's exact location. Deep breathing, coughing, or movement is usually quite painful. There may or may not be a rib deformity, bruise, or laceration of the area. Shortness of breath, severe coughing, or coughing up blood all indicate a major injury rather than a simple rib fracture.

Do *not* bind, strap, or tape a rib fracture. Such wrapping predisposes the victim to pneumonia. Instead, the victim can hold a pillow against the injured area. Instruct the victim to take deep breaths to prevent pneumonia. With multiple rib fractures, the victim may be more comfortable with the arm strapped to the chest with a sling and several swathes.

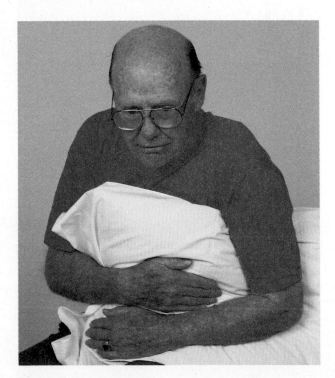

Pillow over broken ribs

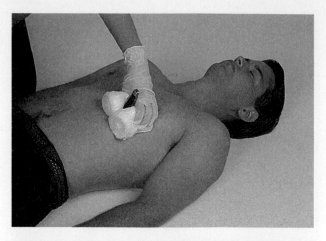

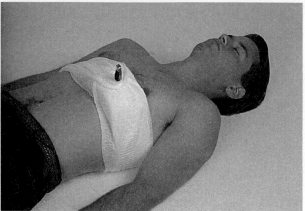

Stabilizing impaled object

Flail chest. A rib fracture involving three or more adjacent ribs that are broken in more than one place is known as a **flail chest** and represents a serious injury. The chest wall may move in the opposite direction to the rest of the chest wall during breathing (called **paradoxical breathing**). Stabilize the ribs by holding a pillow against them to improve breathing. Place the victim in a semisitting position, inclined to the injured side to assist breathing.

Penetrating wound. This wound must be closed quickly to prevent outside air from entering the chest cavity. Do *not* remove or attempt to remove an impaled object because bleeding and air in the chest cavity can occur. Stabilize the object in place with bulky dressings and pads.

A **sucking chest wound** can occur. Have the victim take a breath and let it out; then seal the wound with anything available to stop air from entering the chest cavity. A household plastic wrap folded several times works well, or you can use your hand. Be sure that the wrap is several inches wider than the wound. Place a dressing over the plastic wrap, and tape it in place, leaving one corner untaped. This creates a flutter valve that prevents air from being trapped in the chest cavity. If the victim has trouble breathing, remove the plastic cover to let all air escape, then reapply.

■ CHEST INJURIES ■

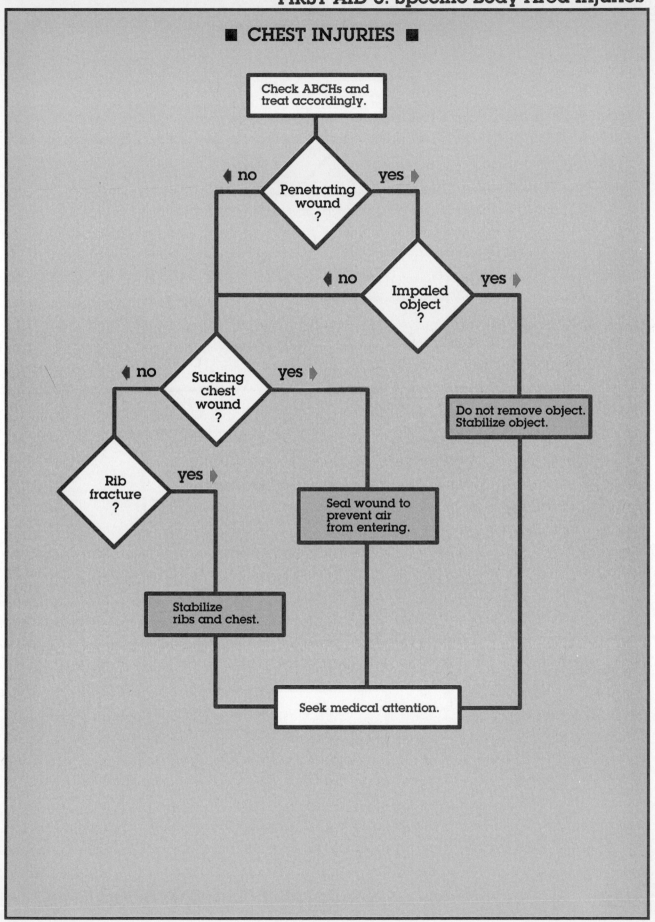

Check ABCHs and treat accordingly.

Penetrating wound ?

no / yes

Impaled object ?

no / yes

Do not remove object. Stabilize object.

Sucking chest wound ?

no / yes

Seal wound to prevent air from entering.

Rib fracture ?

yes

Stabilize ribs and chest.

Seek medical attention.

■ ABDOMINAL INJURIES ■

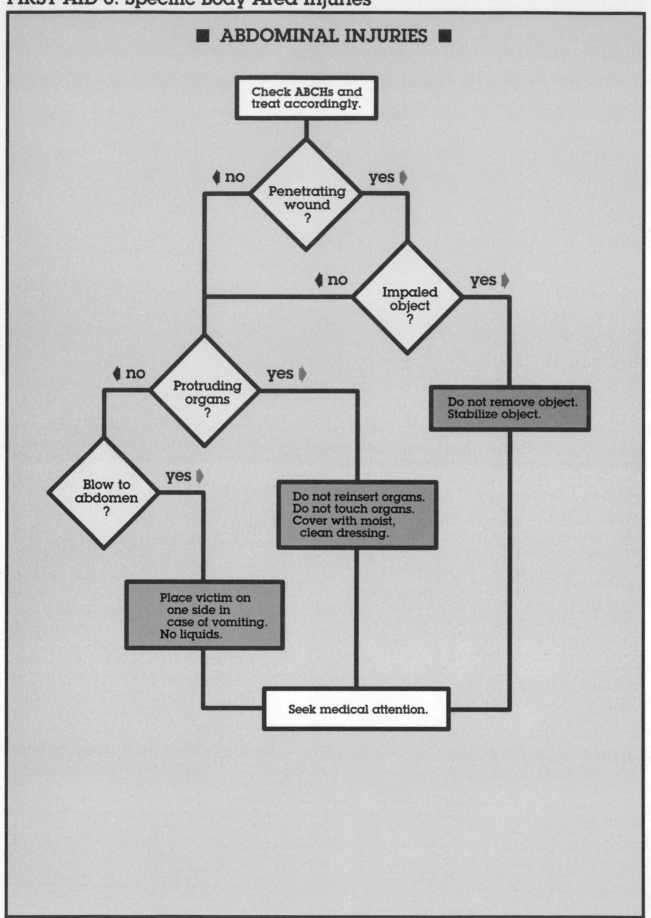

Abdominal Injuries

Abdominal injuries may be **open** or **closed**. **Open injuries** occur when a foreign object enters the abdomen, resulting in external bleeding. **Closed injuries** result from a severe blow that shows no open wound or bleeding on the outside of the body.

Hollow organ (e.g., stomach, intestines) ruptures spill their contents into the abdominal cavity, causing inflammation. Solid organ (e.g., liver, pancreas) ruptures result in severe bleeding.

Signs and Symptoms

- Pain in the abdomen, which may involve cramping
- Legs drawn up to the chest
- Skin wounds and penetrations
- Nausea and vomiting
- Protruding organs
- Blood in the urine or stool
- Guarding abdomen
- Rapid pulse
- Moist, cold skin

Types of Abdominal Injuries and First Aid

Blunt wound. Internal organ bruising and damage can result from a severe blow to the abdomen. Place the victim on one side in a comfortable position, and expect vomiting. Do *not* give liquids or food. Ice chips or sips of water may be given if you are hours from medical assistance.

Penetrating injuries. Expect internal organs to be damaged. If the penetrating object is still in place, leave it in and bandage around it to control external bleeding and to stabilize the object. Do *not* remove the object. Place the victim on his or her side.

Protruding organs. If any of the abdominal organs lie outside the abdominal cavity, do *not* try to replace them inside the abdomen because this introduces infection and could damage the intestine. Keep any extruding organs moist, warm, and clean with a moist, sterile dressing. Do *not* cover them tightly or with any material that clings or disintegrates when wet. Place the victim on his or her side.

Finger and Toe Injuries

Hands and feet are marvels of complexity that are able to sustain considerable abuse. Nevertheless, fingers and toes are often injured.

Fractures

The presence of swelling and tenderness help identify a fractured finger. However, one of the most useful ways to tell if a finger might be broken is by using

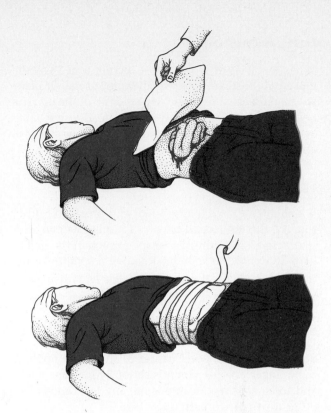

Protruding organs. Do not reinsert them. Cover them with a moist sterile dressing.

the "tapping" test. In this test the victim holds the fingers in full extension. The first aider firmly taps the ends of the victim's fingers toward the victim's hand, transmitting the force down the shaft of the finger's bones and producing pain if a fracture is present. If this tapping produces additional pain, suspect a broken bone. Immobilize the finger by either taping the injured finger to an adjacent finger or by following the procedures described on page 80.

Dislocations

The victim of a dislocated finger often attempts to pull the joint back in place. This is not recommended. The dislocation should be reduced by a physician after x-rays are taken to see that no other injury is involved. Care for the finger as you would a fracture.

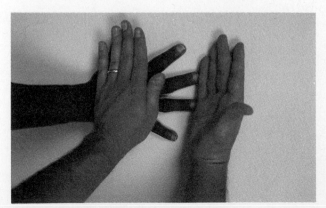

Tapping or percussion test

Nail Avulsion

When a nail is partly torn loose, do not trim away the loose nail. Instead, secure the damaged nail in place with an adhesive bandage. If part or all of the nail has been completely torn away, apply an adhesive bandage coated with antibiotic ointment. A new nail will appear about a month or so later.

Splinters

If a splinter passes under a nail and breaks off flush, remove the embedded part by grasping its end with tweezers after cutting a V-shaped notch in the nail to gain access to the splinter. Remove a splinter in the skin by teasing it out with a sterile needle until the end can be grasped with tweezers or fingers.

Bleeding and Wounds

Standard first aid (see Chapter 5) should be applied. Take finger and toe wounds seriously because nerve and tendon damage can accompany lacerations and other types of wounds.

Amputations

Fingers and toes are the body parts most often amputated. Standard first aid (see Chapter 5) should be applied.

Bandaging/Splinting

Place an injured hand into what is called the "position of function" (finger joints flexed as you would when comfortably holding a baseball). A wad of bulky dressings and cloths is then placed in the palm of the hand. Apply to the palm side of the hand and secure with a roller bandage either a padded board splint or about 40 pages of folded newspapers.

Bleeding Under a Fingernail

Blood can collect under a fingernail after any direct blow to the fingernail. The accumulated blood under the nail causes severe pain.

First Aid

- Immerse the end of the finger in ice water or apply an ice pack against the injured nail.
- Relieve the severe pain by one of two methods:

    1. Using a rotary action, drill through the nail with the sharp point of a knife. This method can produce pain.

    2. Straighten the end of a metal (noncoated) wire paper clip. Hold the paper clip by pliers

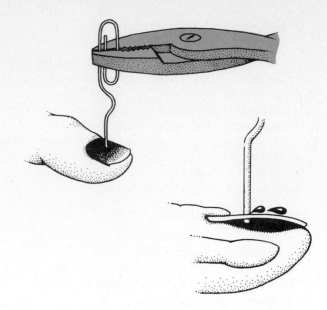

Making a hole in a fingernail

and heat the paper clip until red-hot (best done with a match). Press the glowing end of the clip to the nail so it melts through. Little pressure is needed. The nail has no nerves, so this causes no pain.

- Apply a dressing to absorb the draining blood and to protect the injured nail.

Fishhook Removal

Tape an embedded fishhook in place and do *not* try to remove it if injury to a nearby body part (e.g., eye) or an underlying structure (e.g., blood vessel or nerve) is possible, or if the victim is uncooperative.

If only the point and not the barb of a fishhook penetrates the skin, remove the fishhook by backing it out. Then treat the wound like a puncture wound and seek medical attention for a possible tetanus shot.

However, if the hook's barb has entered the skin, follow these procedures:

1. If medical care is near, transport the victim and have a physician remove the hook.

2. If in a remote area far from medical care, remove the hook by either the pliers method or the fishline method.

Pliers Method ("push and cut")

- Pliers must have tempered jaws that can cut through a hook. The proper kind of pliers is usually unavailable or the barb is buried too deeply to be pushed through. Test the pliers by first cutting a similar fishhook.
- Use cold or hard pressure around the hook to provide temporary numbness.

- Push the embedded hook further in, in a shallow curve, until the point and barb come out through the skin.
- Cut the barb off and back the hook out the way it came in.
- After removing the hook, treat the wound and seek medical attention for a possible tetanus shot.

Fishline Method ("push and pull")

- Loop a piece of fishline over the bend or curve of the embedded hook.
- Stabilize the victim's hooked body area.
- Use cold or hard pressure around the hook to provide temporary numbness.
- With one hand, press down on the hook's shank and eye while the other hand sharply jerks the fishline that is over the hook's bend or curve. The jerk movement should be parallel to the skin's surface. The hook will neatly come out of the same hole it entered, causing little pain.
- After removing the hook, treat the wound and seek medical attention for a possible tetanus shot.

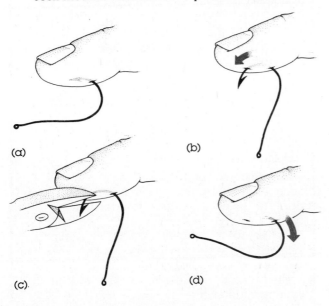

(a) (b)

(c) (d)

Fishhook removal: pliers method

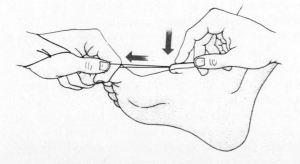

Fishhook removal: fishline method

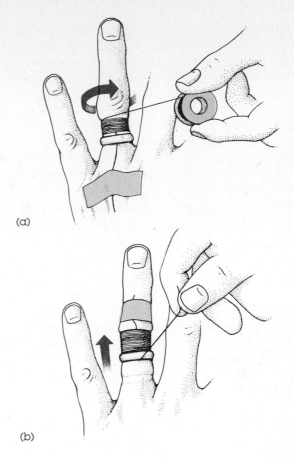

(a)

(b)

Ring removal with string

Ring Removal

Sometimes a finger is too swollen for a ring to be removed. Ring strangulation can be a serious problem if it cuts off circulation long enough. Gangrene may result within four or five hours. Try one or more of the following methods:

1. Lubricate the finger with grease, oil, butter, petroleum jelly, or some other slippery substance, then try to remove the ring.

2. Immerse the finger in cold water for several minutes to reduce the swelling.

3. Massage the finger from the tip to the hand to move the swelling; lubricate the finger again and try removing the ring.

4. Slide several inches of thin string under the ring toward the hand. Push the string under the ring with a match stick or toothpick. Then wrap the string tightly around the finger below the ring, going toward the fingernail and away from the ring. Each wrap should be right next to the one before. While holding the wrapping snugly in place with the fingers of one hand, grasp the upper end of the string with the other hand. Pull the string downward over the ring. The ring may slide over the string. Repeat the procedure several times to get the ring off.

5. Start about an inch from the ring edge and smoothly wind string around the finger, going toward the ring with one strand touching the next. Continue winding smoothly and tightly right up to the edge of the ring. The advantage of this method is that it tends to push the swelling toward the hand. Slip the string end under the ring with a match stick or toothpick. Slowly unwind the string on the hand side of the ring. You should then be able to gently twist the ring off the finger over the wound and string.

6. Cut the narrowest part of the ring with a ring saw, jeweler's saw, ring cutter, or fine hacksaw blade. Protect the exposed portions of the finger.

7. Inflate an ordinary balloon (preferably a slender, tube-shaped one) about three-fourths full. Tie the end. Insert the victim's swollen finger into the end of the balloon so that the balloon rolls back evenly around the finger. In about 15 minutes, the finger should return to its normal size and the ring can be removed.

Blisters

A blister is a collection of fluid in a "bubble" under the outer layer of skin. If not infected, blisters usually heal in three to seven days.

Signs and Symptoms

- Fluid collection under the skin's outer layer
- Pain resulting from touch or pressure
- Swelling and redness around the blister

First Aid

After a blister forms, prevent further injury and reduce pain from pressure by covering small blisters with an adhesive bandage. A large blister should be covered with a porous, plastic-coated gauze pad (which allows the area to breathe) or a stack of gauze pads cut in a doughnut shape to dissipate pressure from the blister. Whenever possible, do *not* break a blister.

When a blister must be broken because of pain:

- Wash the area with soap and warm water. Dry and swab the area with 70% rubbing alcohol.
- Make several small holes at the base of the blister with a sterilized needle. Sterilize the needle by either soaking it in rubbing alcohol or holding it until it gets red over the top of a match flame. Let it cool before using.
- Drain the fluid by gently pressing the blister's top. Do *not* remove the blister's roof. In some cases, the blister may have to be drained several times in the first 24 hours. Apply an antibiotic ointment over the site and cover with a sterile dressing to protect the area from further irritation. After several days, "unroof" any dead

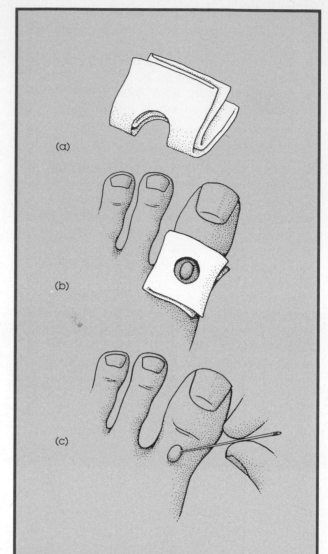

Blister Care a. For an unbroken blister, cut holes in several gauze pads. **b.** Stack the pads on the skin with the holes over the blister. Loosely tape an uncut gauze pad over the top. **c.** If blister is painful or likely to break, puncture the blister's edge with a sterilized needle. Drain all the fluid. Tape a sterile or clean gauze pad or cloth over the flattened blister.

skin by using tweezers to lift the skin, and cut it away with scissors. Reapply antibiotic ointment and a sterile gauze dressing.

- If a blister has ruptured and its roof is gone, apply antibiotic ointment, a sterile gauze dressing, and stacked sterile dressings cut in a doughnut shape. All ruptured blisters should be cleaned with soap and water to prevent infection.
- Check daily for signs of infection (redness or pus). See a doctor if the blister becomes infected. These procedures apply only to friction blisters—*not* to blisters formed from burns, frostbite, or contact with poisonous plants.

■ FISHHOOK REMOVAL ■

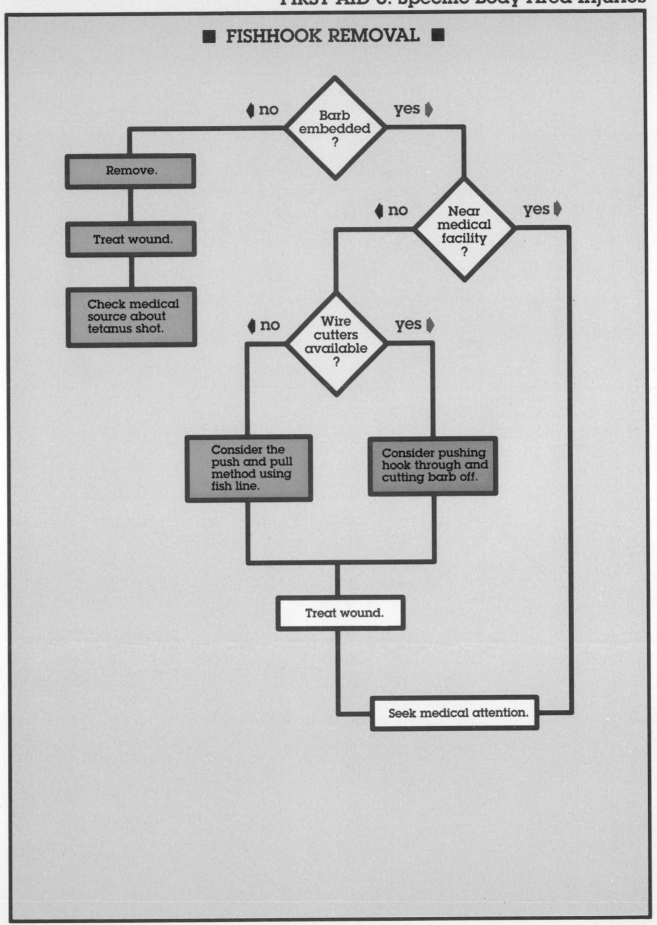

no ◄ **Barb embedded ?** yes ►

Remove.

Treat wound.

Check medical source about tetanus shot.

no ◄ **Near medical facility ?** yes ►

no ◄ **Wire cutters available ?** yes ►

Consider the push and pull method using fish line.

Consider pushing hook through and cutting barb off.

Treat wound.

Seek medical attention.

■ BLISTERS ■

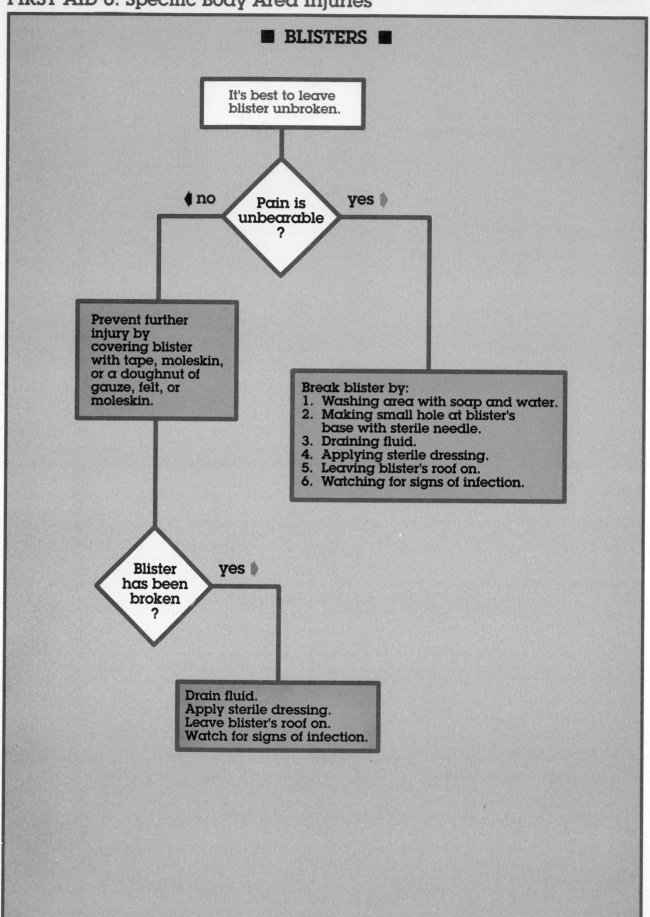

It's best to leave blister unbroken.

Pain is unbearable?

no → Prevent further injury by covering blister with tape, moleskin, or a doughnut of gauze, felt, or moleskin.

yes → Break blister by:
1. Washing area with soap and water.
2. Making small hole at blister's base with sterile needle.
3. Draining fluid.
4. Applying sterile dressing.
5. Leaving blister's roof on.
6. Watching for signs of infection.

Blister has been broken?

yes → Drain fluid.
Apply sterile dressing.
Leave blister's roof on.
Watch for signs of infection.

■ ACTIVITY 1 ■
Head Injury

Check (✓) the signs and symptoms of a skull fracture.

1. _____ Pain at the injury site
2. _____ Deformed skull
3. _____ Fluid leaking from ears or nose
4. _____ Discoloration around eye(s) (black eyes)
5. _____ Pupil of one eye larger than pupil of the other eye

Mark each sign yes (Y) or no (N).

After a head injury, which signs indicate a need for medical attention?

1. _____ Headache lasting more than a day or increased severity
2. _____ Vomiting beginning hours after the initial injury
3. _____ One pupil appearing larger than the other
4. _____ Convulsions or seizures
5. _____ "Seeing double"

■ ACTIVITY 2 ■
Eye Injury

Mark each action yes (Y) or no (N).

Which represents proper first aid for an embedded object in the eye?

1. _____ Using a damp, sterile or clean cloth to remove an object lying on an eyeball's surface
2. _____ Using a toothpick, match stick, etc., to remove a foreign object
3. _____ For an embedded object, using a paper cup or similar item over the eye but not touching the object
4. _____ Allowing the victim to see by leaving the uninjured eye uncovered

Mark each action yes (Y) or no (N).

If a tree limb scrapes against an eye and cuts the eyeball, first aid, besides seeking medical help for the victim, includes:

1. _____ Applying a dressing tightly over the injured eye
2. _____ Holding the eyelids of the injured eye open
3. _____ Applying direct pressure to the cut eyeball in order to control the bleeding
4. _____ Loosely applying dressings over both eyes
5. _____ Tightly applying a dressing over both eyes

Mark each statement true (T) or false (F).

1. _____ Hitting the eye may cause a black eye.
2. _____ An ophthalmologist should see blurred vision victims.
3. _____ For an eyeball knocked out of socket, gently and carefully replace the eyeball in the socket and cover with a dressing.
4. _____ After a blow to the eye apply a cold compress immediately for about 15 minutes to reduce pain and swelling.

Choose the best answer.

1. _____ Corrosive acid has spilled into a coworker's eyes, resulting in severe pain. What should you do first?
   A. Cover both eyes with dressings and immediately obtain medical aid.
   B. Hold eyes open and flood them with water for 15 minutes.
   C. Allow tears to flush out the chemicals.
   D. Pour water into eyes for about 5 minutes.

2. ___ Following your initial actions, which one should you do?
A. Place wet dressings over both eyes.
B. Leave both eyes uncovered and seek medical attention.
C. Allow the victim to rest for at least 30 minutes.
D. Apply dressings over both eyes and seek medical attention.

3. ___ A welder suffers ultraviolet light eye burns. Which first aid procedure does not apply?
A. Apply cold, wet dressings.
B. Have the victim rest with eyes closed.
C. Do not cover the eyes.
D. Seek medical attention.

■ ACTIVITY 3 ■
Nosebleeds

Choose the best techniques for controlling most nosebleeds.

1. ___ A. Position victim in a sitting position.
B. Position victim lying down.

2. ___ A. Keep the head tilted or slightly backward.
B. Keep the head tilted slightly forward.

3. ___ A. Pinch both nostrils for 5 minutes.
B. Pinch only one nostril for 60 seconds.

4. ___ A. Always seek medical attention.
B. Seek medical attention for those taking blood thinners, large doses of aspirin, or those with high blood pressure.

■ ACTIVITY 4 ■
Dental Injuries

Mark each statement true (T) or false (F).

1. ___ Use dental floss rather than a toothpick to remove an object stuck between teeth.

2. ___ If a tooth is knocked out, attempt reimplantation (placing tooth back in the socket) if you are in a remote area with no dentists nearby.

3. ___ Clean and scrub the tooth before attempting to reimplant.

4. ___ Put the knocked-out tooth in mouthwash or alcohol to preserve it.

■ ACTIVITY 5 ■
Chest Injuries

Mark each statement yes (Y) or no (N).

1. Which of the following actions serve as effective immediate first aid for a sucking chest wound?
A. ___ Remove a penetrating object from the chest.
B. ___ Apply a sterile or clean dressing loosely over the wound.
C. ___ Leave the wound uncovered.
D. ___ Tape a piece of plastic tightly over the wound.

Check (✓) the appropriate action(s).

2. If the victim has trouble breathing after you have taped a piece of plastic over a sucking chest wound, you should:
A. ___ Apply a second piece of plastic over the first.
B. ___ Remove the plastic covering from the wound to allow air to escape from the chest cavity and then reapply.
C. ___ Leave the plastic in place and check breathing.

Complete the following statements.

1. ____ The aim of first aid for a sucking chest wound is to:
   A. Not cover the wound.
   B. Cover the chest's hole immediately to prevent air from entering the chest.

2. ____ The aim of first aid for a flail chest is to:
   A. Stabilize the injured chest wall.
   B. Not bind the injured chest since binding interferes with breathing.

Choose the best answer.

1. ____ Which of the following materials, when taped at the edges, would make an effective covering for a sucking chest wound?
   A. Clear plastic wrap
   B. A large gauze dressing
   C. A wash cloth
   D. A pillow case

2. ____ Flail chest signs and symptoms include:
   A. Blood oozing from the injury site
   B. Pain when breathing
   C. Neck injury
   D. Abnormal movement of part of the chest wall during breathing

■ ACTIVITY 6 ■
Abdominal Injuries

Choose the best answer.

Which is proper first aid for a blow to the abdomen? You suspect internal injuries.

1. ____ A. Place the victim on his or her back with a support on the abdomen.
   B. Place the victim on his or her side.

2. ____ A. Give the victim ice chips or sips of water to drink.
   B. Give the victim nothing to eat or drink.

Select the best first aid choice for a victim's abdominal open wound resulting from a penetrating object.

3. ____ A. Remove the penetrating object.
   B. Leave object in place and stabilize it.

When protruding organs appear through an abdominal wound, you should

4. ____ A. Gently push the organs back into the abdomen
   B. Not attempt to push them back into the abdomen

5. ____ A. Cover the wound with a clean, moist dressing
   B. Cover the wound with a cotton dressing

■ ACTIVITY 7 ■
Finger Injuries

Check the appropriate answer(s).

Relieve the painful pressure caused by the accumulation of blood under a fingernail or toenail by:

1. ____ Placing the finger in hot water for several minutes
2. ____ Drilling a hole through the nail with the point of a knife
3. ____ Melting a hole through the nail to the site of the blood with a red-hot paper clip

Mark each technique yes (Y) or no (N).

Which techniques can be useful in removing a stuck ring?

1. ____ Lubricate the finger with oil, butter, or other slippery substance
2. ____ Place the finger in hot water for several minutes.
3. ____ Use string wrapped tightly around the finger.
4. ____ Cut the ring with a fine-toothed hacksaw.
5. ____ Cut the skin along the ring to relieve pressure.

■ ACTIVITY 8 ■
Blisters

Choose the best answer.

1. ____ After a blister forms, what should be tried first?
   A. Drain the blister by making a small hole at the blister's edge.
   B. Use scissors to remove the blister's top.
   C. Cover with gauze or tape cut into the shape of a doughnut.

2. ____ When can a blister be broken?
   A. When very painful
   B. At least three days after its appearance
   C. Never by a first aider

3. ____ Which is the proper procedure for breaking a blister?
   A. Cut the entire roof of the blister off.
   B. Drain the fluid by making a small hole at the blister's edge.
   C. Use a red-hot paper clip to puncture the skin.
   D. Pinch or squeeze the blister off.
   E. Soak the blister off in hot water.
   F. None of these, since blisters should never be broken.

7

Poisoning

■ Swallowed Poison ■ Insect Stings ■ Snakebites ■ Spider Bites ■ Scorpion Stings ■
■ Tick Removal ■ Poison Ivy, Oak and Sumac ■ Carbon Monoxide ■

A poison is a relatively small amount of any substance (solid, liquid, or gas) that when swallowed, inhaled, absorbed, or injected can by its chemical action damage tissue or adversely change organ function and thus can affect health or cause death.

Swallowed Poison

Deaths by swallowing poison have dramatically decreased in recent years, particularly in children under age five. Despite this reduction, nonfatal poisoning remains a major cause of hospital admissions and emergency room care. For every poisoning death among children under the age of five, 80,000 to 90,000 nonfatal cases are seen in emergency rooms and about 20,000 children are hospitalized.

Signs and Symptoms

- Abdominal pain and cramping
- Nausea or vomiting
- Diarrhea
- Burns, odor, stains around and in mouth
- Drowsiness or unconsciousness
- Poison containers or plants nearby

First Aid

- Determine the critical information, which includes:
    1. *Who?* Age and size of the victim
    2. *What?* Type of poison swallowed
    3. *How much?* A taste, half a bottle, etc.
    4. *How?* Circumstances
    5. *When?* Time taken
- Contact the poison control center, hospital emergency department, or a physician immediately. Some poisons produce little damage until hours later, while others do damage immediately. More than 70% of poisonings can be treated through instructions taken over the telephone. Otherwise, victims should be transported to a medical facility.
- Check respirations and pulse often, if victim is unconscious.

- Unless a medical authority advises it, do *not* automatically give water or milk to dilute except when the victim has swallowed caustics or corrosives (e.g., acids and alkalis). Reasons include the fact that fluids may dissolve tablets or capsules more rapidly, and may fill up the stomach, thus forcing poison into the small intestines where absorption is faster. Use water instead of milk whenever possible in case syrup of ipecac is used later because the milk may bind the ipecac and delay vomiting.
- Do *not* induce vomiting unless a medical authority advises it. Inducing vomiting removes 30–50% of the poison from the stomach. Inducing vomiting must be done within 30 minutes of swallowing or before the poison leaves the stomach.

A medical authority will usually say *never* induce vomiting for:

- A victim with seizures
- An unconscious or drowsy victim
- A woman in the late stages of pregnancy
- A person with a history of advanced heart disease or who is likely to suffer a heart attack
- A person who has swallowed corrosives (strong acids and alkalis)
- A victim who has swallowed petroleum products (e.g., gasoline, lighter fluid, furniture polish)
- A person who has swallowed strychnine
- A child less than 6 months old

Do *not* use salt water to induce vomiting because it is dangerous and can kill children. Do *not* gag the victim by sticking a finger down his or her throat since it is usually ineffective in causing vomiting (only in 15% of cases does it work) and it wastes time.

Many poisons induce vomiting for some victims; others require syrup of ipecac. It can be purchased without a prescription, and is easily given, effective, and relatively safe.

If instructed by a medical authority to induce vomiting by using syrup of ipecac, give:

- Adults: 2 tablespoons with 2–3 glasses of water

■ SWALLOWED POISON ■

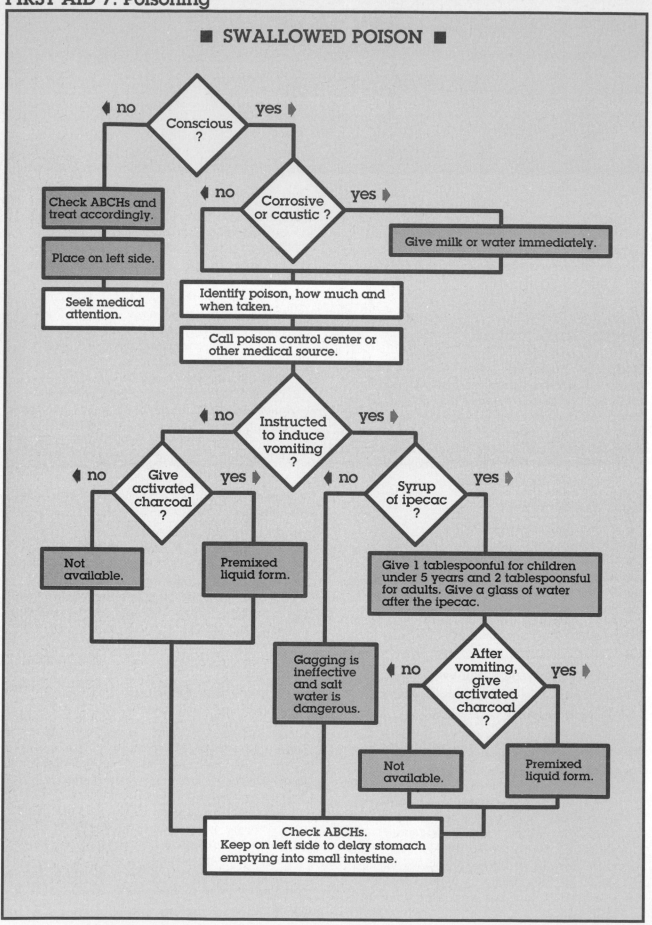

How to Poison-Proof Your Home

1. Keep all medicines (including over-the-counter products), cleaning products, automotive care products and plants out of reach of children. Store them up high or in locked cabinets.

2. Use products with child-resistant packaging and always replace the cap properly. But don't rely on the packaging alone to protect your child.

3. Use medicines wisely. Follow label or prescription instructions carefully. Give prescription medicine only to the person for whom it was prescribed. Discard outdated medications safely—flush them down the toilet, rinse out the container and bury it deep in the trash.

4. Avoid transferring poisonous products from their original containers. If you must do this, carefully copy all information from the original label—product name, expiration date, contents—and attach it to the new container. And never put poisonous substances into a container that once held food, such as a soda bottle. Even an adult may mistake the contents for an edible product.

5. Store harmful products away from food, and store external medications separately from internal medications to lessen the chance of someone mistaking one for the other.

6. Do not refer to medicine as ''candy'' when talking to children—they may take you literally. And don't take medicine in front of the children. Their imitative behavior may lead to tragedy.

7. Keep a one-ounce bottle of syrup of ipecac to induce vomiting for each child in the house, but don't administer it without professional medical advice. (Syrup of ipecac is available from your pharmacist.) Keep the number of your local poison control center, hospital emergency room or family doctor posted near the phone.

Source: National Safety Council, Family Safety & Health.

- Children: 1 tablespoon with 1–2 glasses of water
- Infants: 1–2 teaspoons with 1 bottle or glass of water (when possible, infants should be given ipecac in a medical facility)

Syrup of ipecac may take up to 20 minutes to work. Vomiting occurs in 97% of all people and a second dose is seldom needed. However, repeat the initial dosage once if the victim does not vomit after 20 minutes.

- Activated charcoal can be given after the victim has stopped vomiting. This substance handles the remaining poison in the stomach since syrup of ipecac removes only 30–50% of swallowed poisons. Activated charcoal acts like a sponge and binds the poison within the digestive system. Substances such as burned toast, fireplace ashes, and charcoal briquettes are all ineffective. Most pharmacies do not routinely carry activated charcoal. First aiders seldom give it since a victim can usually arrive at a medical facility within minutes.
- Save poison containers, plants, and vomit to help medical personnel identify the poison and prescribe appropriate treatment.
- Position unconscious victims on their side and do *not* give anything by mouth.
- Do *not* follow a container label's first aid procedures or recommended antidotes without getting confirmation from a medical authority since many labels are wrong.

Insect Stings

For a severely allergic person, a single sting may be fatal within 15 minutes. Although accounts exist of individuals who have survived some 2,000 stings, 500 or more stings will kill most people who are not allergic to stinging insects.

Some experts report that 1% of all children and 4% of adults have such an allergy. An estimated 50–100 sting-related deaths occur yearly. The number of cases

Avoiding Insect Stings

Here are some ways to avoid being stung:

1. Have a nonallergic person destroy any insect nests that appear around the home or yard.

2. Do not go barefoot or wear sandals outdoors.

3. Wear close-fitting clothes that won't trap an insect. Long-sleeved shirts, long pants, and gloves provide protection. They should be light-weight for comfort on hot days.

4. Do not look or smell like a flower. Brightly colored clothing, perfumed lotions, aftershaves, shampoos, and cosmetics can attract insects.

5. Be alert while eating outdoors since food and garbage attract insects.

6. If you find yourself close to an insect, do not swat or run since such actions can trigger an attack. Retreat slowly, or if retreat is impossible, lie face down and cover your head with your arms.

may actually be higher but not reported as involving insect stings because they are mistaken for heart attacks or naturally caused death.

Signs and Symptoms

- **Usual reactions.** Momentary pain, redness around sting site, itching, heat

- **Worrisome reactions.** Skin flush, hives, localized swelling of lips or tongue, "tickle" in throat, wheezing, abdominal cramps, diarrhea
- **Life-threatening reactions.** Bluish or grayish skin color (cyanosis), seizures, unconsciousness, inability to breathe due to swelling of vocal cords

TABLE 7-1 Facts About Troublesome Insects

Description	Habitat	Problem	Severity	Treatment	Protection
Chigger Oval with red velvety covering. Sometimes almost colorless. Larva has six legs. Harmless adult has eight and resembles a small spider. Very tiny— about 1/20-inch long.	Found in low damp places covered with vegetation: shaded woods, high grass or weeds, fruit orchards. Also lawns and golf courses. From Canada to Argentina.	Attaches itself to the skin by inserting mouthparts into a hair follicle. Injects a digestive fluid that causes cells to disintegrate. Then feeds on cell parts. It does not suck blood.	Itching from secreted enzymes results several hours after contact. Small red welts appear. Secondary infection often follows. Degree of irritation varies with individuals.	Lather with soap and rinse several times to remove chiggers. If welts have formed, dab antiseptic on area. Severe lesions may require antihistamine ointment.	Apply proper repellent to clothing, particularly near uncovered areas such as wrists and ankles. Apply to skin. Spray or dust infested areas (lawns, plants) with suitable chemicals.
Bedbug Flat oval body with short broad head and six legs. Adult is reddish brown. Young are yellowish white. Unpleasant pungent odor. From 1/8- to 1/4-inch in length.	Hides in crevices, mattresses, under loose wallpaper during day. At night travels considerable distance to find victims. Widely distributed throughout the world.	Punctures the skin with piercing organs and sucks blood. Local inflammation and welts result from anticoagulant enzyme that bug secretes from salivary glands while feeding.	Affects people differently. Some have marked swelling and considerable irritation; others aren't bothered. Sometimes transmits serious diseases.	Apply antiseptic to prevent possible infection. Bug usually bites sleeping victim, gorges itself completely in 3 to 5 minutes and departs. It's rarely necessary to remove one.	Spray beds, mattresses, bed springs, and baseboards with insecticide. Bugs live in large groups. They migrate to new homes on water pipes and clothing.
Brown Recluse Spider Oval body with eight legs. Light yellow to medium dark brown. Has distinctive mark shaped like a fiddle on its back. Body from 3/8- to 1/2-inch long, 1/4-inch wide, 3/4-inch from toe-to-toe.	Prefers dark places where it's seldom disturbed. Outdoors: old trash piles, debris, and rough ground. Indoors: attics, storerooms, closets. Found in southern and midwestern United States.	Bites produce an almost painless sting that may not be noticed, at first. Shy, it bites only when annoyed or surprised. Left alone, it won't bite. Victim rarely sees the spider.	In 2 to 8 hours pain may be noticed, followed by blisters, swelling, hemorrhage, or ulceration. Some people experience rash, nausea, jaundice, chills, fever, cramps, or joint pain.	Summon doctor. Bite may require hospitalization for a few days. Full healing may take from 6 to 8 weeks. Weak adults and children have been known to die.	Use caution when cleaning secluded areas in the home or using machinery usually left idle. Check firewood, inside shoes, packed clothing and bedrolls— frequent hideaways.
Black Widow Spider Color varies from dark brown to glossy black. Densely covered with short microscopic hairs. Red or yellow hourglass marking on the underside of the female's abdomen. Male does not have this mark and is not poisonous. Overall length with legs extended is 1 1/2 inch. Body is 1/4-inch wide.	Found with eggs and web. Outside: in vacant rodent holes, under stones, logs, in long grass, hollow stumps, and brush piles. Inside: in dark corners of barns, garages, piles of stone, wood. Most bites occur in outhouses. Found in southern Canada, throughout United States, except Alaska.	Bites cause local redness. Two tiny red spots may appear. Pain follows almost immediately. Larger muscles become rigid. Body temperature rises slightly. Profuse perspiration and tendency toward nausea follow. It's usually difficult to breathe or talk. May cause constipation, urine retention.	Venom is more dangerous than a rattlesnake's but is given in much smaller amounts. About 5% of bite cases result in death. Death is from asphyxiation due to respiratory paralysis. More dangerous for children; to adults its worst feature is pain. Convulsions result in some cases.	Use an antiseptic such as alcohol or hydrogen peroxide on the bitten area to prevent secondary infection. Keep victim quiet and call a doctor. Do not treat as you would a snakebite since this will only increase the pain and chance of infection; bleeding will not remove the venom.	Wear gloves when working in areas where there might be spiders. Destroy any egg sacs you find. Spray insecticide in any area where spiders are usually found, especially under privy seats. Check them out regularly. General cleanliness, paint, and light discourage spiders.

TABLE 7-1 Facts About Troublesome Insects (continued)

Description	Habitat	Problem	Severity	Treatment	Protection
Scorpion Crablike appearance with clawlike pincers. Fleshy post-abdomen or "tail" has five segments, ending in a bulbous sac and stinger. Two poisonous types: solid straw yellow or yellow with irregular black stripes on back. From 2 1/2 to 4 inches long.	Spends days under loose stones, bark, boards, floors of outhouses. Burrows in the sand. Roams freely at night. Crawls under doors into homes. Lethal types are found only in the warm desert-like climate of Arizona and adjacent areas.	Stings by thrusting its tail forward over its head. Swelling or discoloration of the area indicates a nondangerous, though painful, sting. A dangerously toxic sting doesn't change the appearance of the area, which does become hypersensitive.	Excessive salivation and facial contortions may follow. Temperature rises to over 104°F. Tongue becomes sluggish. Convulsions, in waves of increasing intensity, may lead to death from nervous exhaustion. First 3 hours most critical.	Apply constriction. Keep victim quiet and call a doctor immediately. Do not cut the skin or give pain killers. They increase the killing power of the venom. Antitoxin, readily available to doctors, has proved to be very effective.	Apply a petroleum distillate to any dwelling places that cannot be destroyed. Cats are considered effective predators, as are ducks and chickens, though the latter are more likely to be stung and killed. Don't go barefoot at night.
Bee Winged body with yellow and black stripes. Covered with branched or feathery hairs. Makes a buzzing sound. Different species vary from 1/2 to 1 inch in length.	Lives in aerial or underground nests or hives. Widely distributed throughout the world wherever there are flowering plants—from the polar regions to the equator.	Stings with tail when annoyed. Burning and itching with localized swelling occur. Usually leaves venom sac in victim. It takes between 2 and 3 minutes to inject all the venom.	If a person is allergic, more serious reactions occur—nausea, shock, unconsciousness. Swelling may occur in another part of the body. Death may result.	Gently scrape (don't pluck) the stinger so venom sac won't be squeezed. Wash with soap and antiseptic. If swelling occurs, contact doctor. Keep victim warm while resting.	Have exterminator destroy nests and hives. Avoid wearing sweet fragrances and bright clothing. Keep food covered. Move slowly or stand still in the vicinity of bees.
Mosquito Small dark fragile body with transparent wings and elongated mouthparts. From 1/8- to 1/4-inch long.	Found in temperate climates throughout the world where the water necessary for breeding is available.	Bites and sucks blood. Itching and localized swelling result. Bite may turn red. Only the female is equipped to bite.	Sometimes transmits yellow fever, malaria, encephalitis, and other diseases. Scratching can cause secondary infections.	Don't scratch. Lather with soap and rinse to avoid infection. Apply antiseptic to relieve itching.	Destroy available breeding water to check multiplication. Place nets on windows and beds. Use proper repellent.
Tarantula Large dark "spider" with a furry covering. From 6 to 7 inches in toe-to-toe diameter.	Found in southwestern United States. The tropical varieties are poisonous.	Bites produce pinprick sensation with negligible effect. It will not bite unless teased.	Usually no more dangerous than a pin prick. Has only local effects.	Wash and apply antiseptic to prevent the possibility of secondary infection.	Harmless to man, the tarantula is beneficial since it destroys harmful insects.
Tick Oval with small head; the body is not divided into definite segments. Grey or brown. Measures from 1/4 to 3/4 inch when mature.	Found in all United States areas and in parts of southern Canada, on low shrubs, grass, and trees. Carried around by both wild and domestic animals.	Attaches itself to the skin and sucks blood. After removal there is danger of infection, especially if the mouthparts are left in the wound.	Sometimes carries and spreads Rocky Mountain spotted fever, Lyme disease, Colorado tick fever. In a few rare cases, causes paralysis until removed.	Gently remove with tweezers so none of the mouthparts are left in skin. Wash with soap and water; apply antiseptic.	Cover exposed parts of body when in tick-infested areas. Use proper repellent. Remove ticks attached to clothes, body. Check neck and hair. Bathe.

Source: National Safety Council, Family Safety, *Spring 1980, pp. 20–21.*

First Aid

Those who have had a reaction to an insect sting should be instructed in self-treatment so they can protect themselves from severe reactions. They should also be advised to purchase a medical alert bracelet or necklace identifying them as insect-allergic.

■ Carefully examine the sting site for a stinger embedded in the skin. The bee is the only stinging insect that leaves its stinger behind. If the stinger is still embedded, it needs to be removed, because it will continue to inject poison for two or three minutes unless removed. Do *not* pull at the stinger directly with

■ INSECT STINGS ■
(Flying Insects)

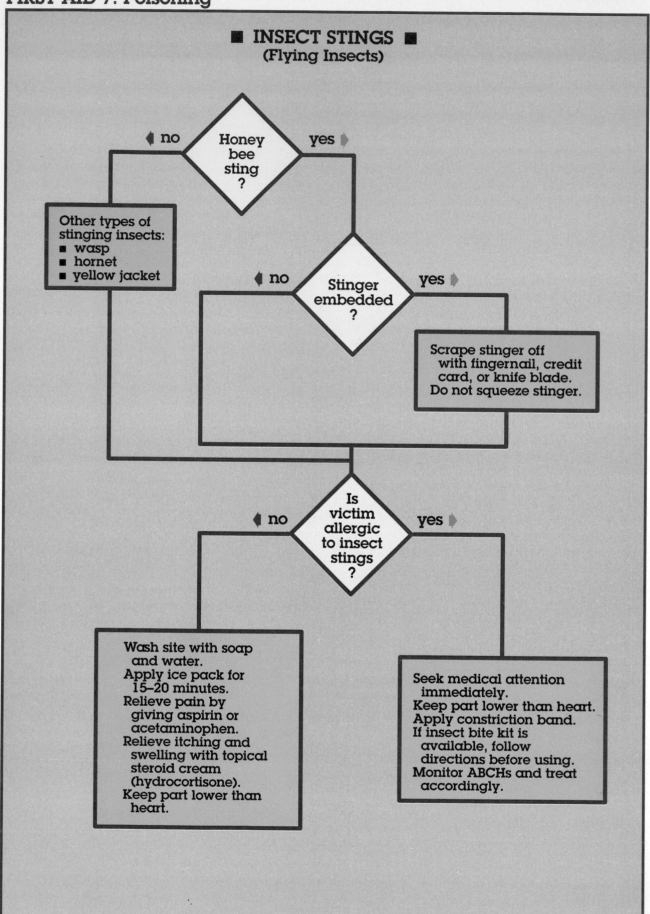

Honey bee sting ?

◀ no   yes ▶

Other types of stinging insects:
- wasp
- hornet
- yellow jacket

Stinger embedded ?

◀ no   yes ▶

Scrape stinger off with fingernail, credit card, or knife blade. Do not squeeze stinger.

Is victim allergic to insect stings ?

◀ no   yes ▶

Wash site with soap and water.
Apply ice pack for 15–20 minutes.
Relieve pain by giving aspirin or acetaminophen.
Relieve itching and swelling with topical steroid cream (hydrocortisone).
Keep part lower than heart.

Seek medical attention immediately.
Keep part lower than heart.
Apply constriction band.
If insect bite kit is available, follow directions before using.
Monitor ABCHs and treat accordingly.

tweezers or fingers because it has a sac at the exposed end that can pump more venom into the victim. Instead scrape the sack away cleanly with a long fingernail, credit card, scissor edge or knife blade.

- Wash the sting site thoroughly.
- Apply an ice pack over the sting site to slow absorption of the venom and relieve pain.
- Several items may help relieve the pain and itching. Because stings are painful, some type of analgesic (e.g., aspirin, acetaminophen) is usually adequate. A topical steroid cream, such as hydrocortisone, may help combat local swelling and itching. An antihistamine may prevent some local symptoms if given early, but it works too slowly to counteract a life-threatening allergic reaction.
- Observe victims for at least 30 minutes for signs of an allergic reaction (anaphylactic shock). For those who are highly allergic, a dose of epinephrine (adrenalin) is the only effective life-saving treatment. It is given subcutaneously at the sting site. A physician can prescribe an emergency kit that includes a prefilled syringe of epinephrine or a spring-loaded device that automatically triggers the injection of epinephrine by a quick thrust into the thigh or large muscle. The spring-loaded device is useful for those reluctant to use a syringe with a visible needle. The allergic person should take the kit whenever going places where stinging insects are known to exist. Refer to the section on anaphylactic shock for more about kits containing epinephrine. Since epinephrine is short-acting, the victim must be watched closely for signs of returning anaphylactic shock, and another dose of epinephrine should be injected as often as

every 15 minutes if needed. Epinephrine should *not* be used to treat a sting unless the victim has an allergic reaction. Epinephrine has a limited shelf life of one to three years, or until it has turned brown.

- Some kits contain an antihistamine. It is *not* an effective emergency treatment and is included in the kit to reduce later symptoms after the epinephrine treatment.
- Some physicians provide their sting-senstitive patients with an inhaler containing epinephrine, and instruct them in its use.

Snakebites

Throughout the world about 50,000 people die each year from snakebite. In the United States, of the 40,000 to 50,000 annually bitten, over 7,000 are bitten by poisonous snakes. Amazingly, less than a dozen Americans die each year. Victims rarely die in the first 24 hours.

Of the many different snake species, only four in the United States are poisonous: rattlesnake, copperhead, water moccasin, and coral snake. The first three are known as pit vipers. They have three common characteristics:

- Triangular, flat head wider than its neck
- Elliptical pupils (i.e., cat's eye)
- Heat-sensitive "pit" located between each eye and nostril

The coral snake is small and very colorful, with a series of bright red, yellow, and black bands around its body. Every other band is yellow. A black snout also marks the coral snake.

Imported snakes, found in zoos, schools, snake farms, and amateur and professional collections, account for at least 15 bites a year. They are smuggled illegally into the U.S. in large numbers.

Pit Vipers

(rattlesnake, copperhead, water moccasin)

Signs and Symptoms

- Severe burning pain at the bite site
- Two small puncture wounds about 1/2 inch apart (some cases may have only one puncture wound)
- Swelling (happens within 5 minutes and can involve an entire extremity)
- Discoloration and blood-filled blisters may develop in 6–10 hours
- In severe cases: nausea, vomiting, sweating, weakness
- No venom injection occurs in about 25% of all poisonous snakebites, only fang and tooth wounds

Fire Ant Bites

Five fire ant species are found in the United States. Particular concern has centered on the imported species, which is more aggressive than the native fire ant. Imported fire ants have become widely distributed in the southern states, from Texas to North Carolina. They have become the most common stinging ants in North America.

The ant bites its victim by securing itself to the skin with its mandibles, causing pain. Then, using its head as a pivot, the ant swings the abdomen in an arc, repeatedly stinging its victim with an abdominal stinger.

The South American fire ants range in color from red to dark brown. They are about 1/8–1/4″ long, and usually live in foot-high, dome-shaped mounds.

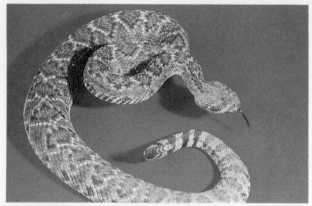

Rattlesnake

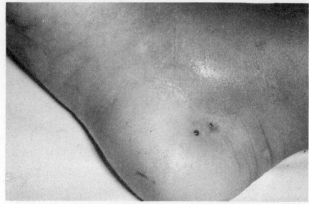

Rattlesnake bite. Note two fang marks.

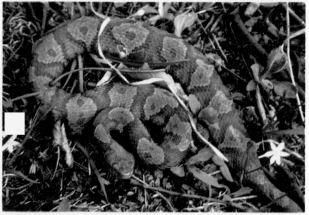

Copperhead snake

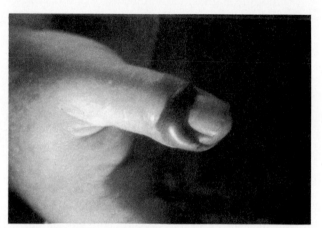

Copperhead bite 2 hours after bite.

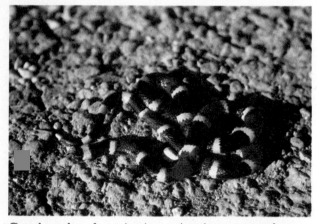

Coral snake. America's most poisonous snake

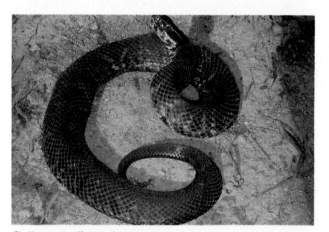

Cottonmouth water moccasin

First Aid

Most snakebites occur within a few hours of a medical facility where antivenin is available. Bites showing no sign of venom injection require only a possible tetanus shot and care of the bite wounds.

Controversy exists about proper first aid procedures for snakebite. The following list represents the most widely accepted first aid procedures:

- Get victim away from snake. Snakes have been known to bite more than once.
- Keep the victim quiet. Do *not* allow victim to increase the heart rate—if possible, transport the victim by carrying. If alone, walk very slowly to help.
- Identify the snake species since snakes vary in their toxicity. This helps in determining the

■ SNAKEBITES ■

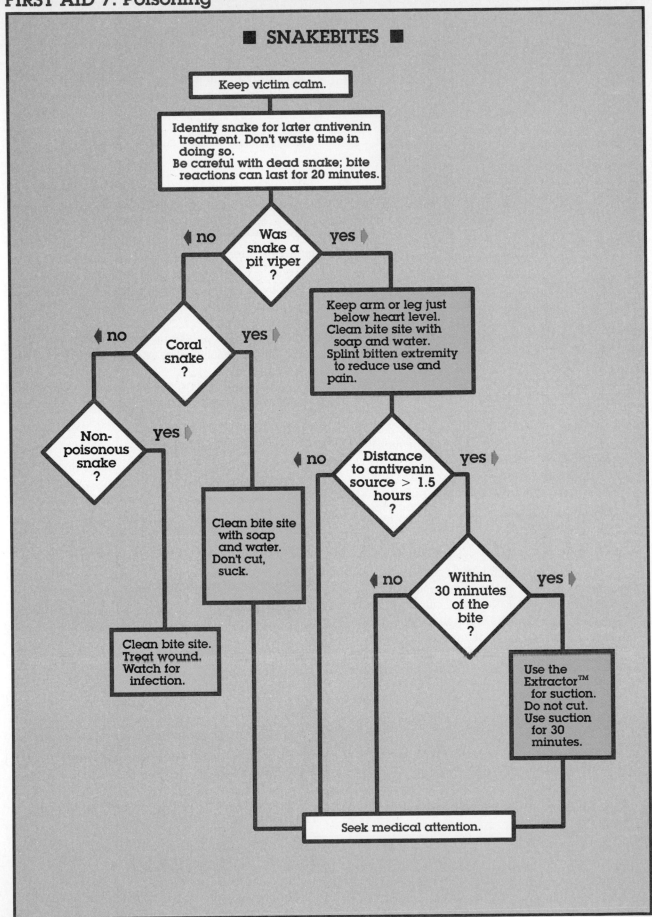

Keep victim calm.

Identify snake for later antivenin treatment. Don't waste time in doing so.
Be careful with dead snake; bite reactions can last for 20 minutes.

Was snake a pit viper?

no → Coral snake?

yes → Keep arm or leg just below heart level. Clean bite site with soap and water. Splint bitten extremity to reduce use and pain.

Coral snake? — no → Non-poisonous snake?

Coral snake? — yes → Clean bite site with soap and water. Don't cut, suck.

Non-poisonous snake? — yes → Clean bite site. Treat wound. Watch for infection.

Distance to antivenin source > 1.5 hours?

yes → Within 30 minutes of the bite?

Within 30 minutes of the bite? — yes → Use the Extractor™ for suction. Do not cut. Use suction for 30 minutes.

Seek medical attention.

amount of antivenin required for treating the victim. Some experts suggest taking the dead snake with the victim to the medical facility. Be careful around a decapitated snake head since head reactions persist for 20 or more minutes.

- Gently wash the bitten area with soap and water.
- Do *not* apply a tourniquet or constriction band.
- Do *not* cut and suck.
- Every 15 minutes keep track of swelling on the victim's skin with a pen and write down the time the mark was made. This shows how rapidly swelling has moved.
- If more than a few hours from a medical facility with antivenin, or if the snake was large and the skin is swelling rapidly, you should apply suction with the Extractor™ immediately. *This procedure is seldom needed because most bites happen within a short distance from medical care.*

If done within the first three minutes of the bite, up to 30% of the venom can be removed, and a lesser amount if done within 30 minutes of the bite. Do *not* apply suction if 30 minutes have passed since the bite. Use the Extractor™ (Sawyer Products) for suction. It does not require an incision (cutting). Apply it within the first 3 minutes of the bite and leave on for 30 minutes.

- Quickly transport all snakebite victims to a medical facility for antivenin. It must be given within 4 hours.
- Do *not* use cold on a snakebite.
- Do *not* use electric shock.

Coral

(not a pit viper snake)

Signs and Symptoms

(apparent after about 1 hour)

- Bite usually happens on a small part of the body (e.g., finger, toe) because of coral's small mouth and teeth. It has to "chew" its venom into the victim.
- One or more punctures or scratchlike wounds
- Little or no local signs (e.g., swelling, discoloration, pain)
- Dizziness, drooling, blurred or double vision, drooping eyelids, drowsiness, nausea, vomiting

First Aid

- Keep victim calm.
- Gently clean bite site with warm soap and water.
- Do *not* apply a constriction band or cut the victim's skin.
- Transport the victim to a medical facility for antivenin.

Nonpoisonous Snakes

Nonpoisonous snakes leave a horseshoe shape of tooth marks on victim's skin.

First Aid

- Gently clean the bitten area with warm soap and water.
- Care for the bite as a minor wound.
- Consult with a medical authority.

Spider Bites

Two spiders, the black widow and the brown recluse, can be deadly.

Black Widow Spider

The black widow spider is found throughout the world. A red spot (often in the shape of an hourglass) on the

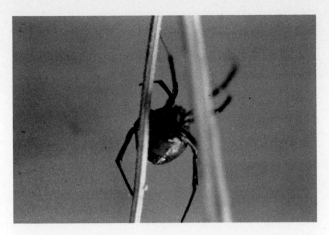

Black widow spider. Note red hourglass configuration on abdomen.

abdomen identifies the female—she is the one that bites. Females have a glossy black body. By volume, black widow spider venom is more deadly than the rattlesnake's, but it is injected in much smaller amounts.

Signs and Symptoms

Determining whether a person has been bitten by a black widow spider is difficult.

- A sharp pinprick of the spider's bite may be felt, although some victims are not even aware of the bite. In no more than 15 minutes a dull, numbing pain develops in the bitten area.
- Faint red bite marks appear.
- Muscle stiffness and cramps occur next, usually affecting the abdomen when the bite is in the lower part of the body or legs, and affecting the shoulders, back, or chest when the bite is on the upper body or arms.
- Headache, chills, fever, heavy sweating, dizziness, nausea, vomiting, and severe abdominal pain afflict the victim.

First Aid

Even without treatment, most healthy adults survive, and few people have died. However, black widow bites can threaten the lives of children and the elderly.

- If possible, catch the spider to confirm its identity. Even if the body is crushed, save it for identification.
- Clean the bitten area with soap and water or alcohol. Do *not* apply a constricting band because the black widow venom's action is swift, and there is little to be gained by trying to slow absorption with a constriction band.
- Place an ice pack over the bite to relieve pain.
- Keep the victim quiet and monitor breathing.
- Seek immediate medical attention. There is an antivenin for black widow bites. It brings relief

of symptoms within one to three hours, especially if given as soon as possible after the victim was bitten. Antivenin use is usually reserved for those under 14 years, older than 65, have hypertension, pregnant, or a severe bite.

Brown Recluse Spider

The brown recluse spider has a brown, possibly purplish, violin-shaped figure on its back. Brown recluse bites are rarely fatal, except for hypersensitive people, children, the elderly, and those with chronic health problems.

Signs and Symptoms

- The initial pain felt may be slight enough to be overlooked.
- A blister at the bite site, along with redness and swelling, appears after several hours.
- Pain, which may remain mild but can become severe, develops within two to eight hours at the bite site.
- Fever, weakness, vomiting, joint pain, and a rash may occur.
- An ulcer forms within a week. Gangrene may develop in some cases.
- Chills, fever, red skin rash, weakness, nausea, and vomiting.

First Aid

1. Pre-ulceration care:
   - If possible, capture the spider for positive identification.
   - Clean the bitten area with alcohol.
   - Apply an ice pack to the bitten area.
   - Seek immediate medical attention.
2. Post-ulceration care:
   - Care for ulcerated wound with Burow's solution.
   - Follow medical advice.

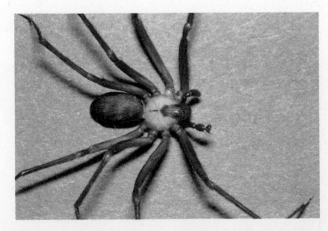

Brown recluse spider. Note violin or fiddle configuration on back.

■ SPIDER BITES AND SCORPION STINGS ■

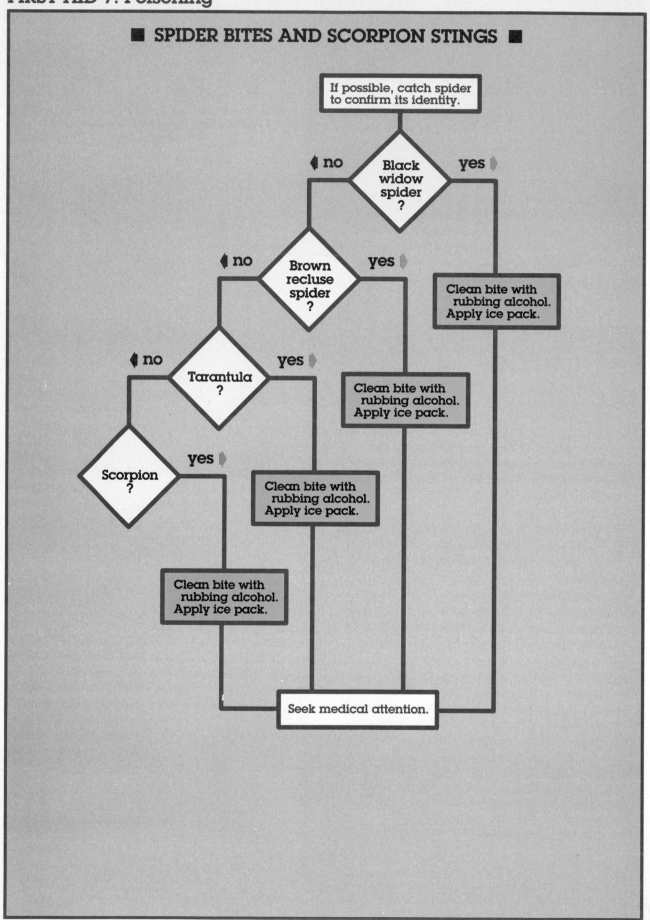

If possible, catch spider to confirm its identity.

Black widow spider ?
no ◄ ► yes

Brown recluse spider ?
no ◄ ► yes

Tarantula ?
no ◄ ► yes

Scorpion ?
► yes

Clean bite with rubbing alcohol. Apply ice pack.

Clean bite with rubbing alcohol. Apply ice pack.

Clean bite with rubbing alcohol. Apply ice pack.

Clean bite with rubbing alcohol. Apply ice pack.

Seek medical attention.

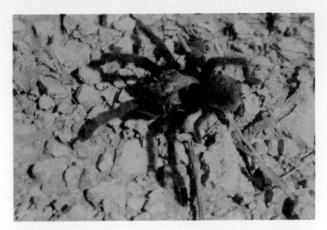

Tarantula

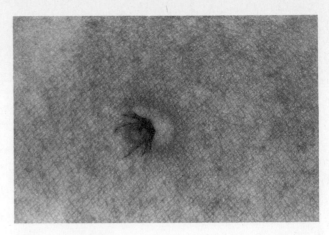

Tick embedded

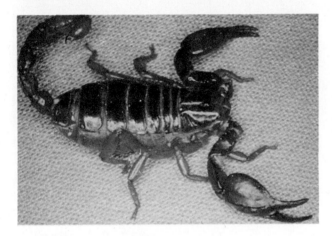

Scorpion

Tarantula Spider

More menacing-looking than black widow and brown recluse spiders, the tarantula rarely produces symptoms other than moderate pain when it bites. First aid involves cleaning the bite wound to prevent infection, placing an ice pack wrapped in a cloth on the bite area, and seeking medical attention.

Scorpion Stings

Death from scorpion stings in the United States is rare; children are at greatest risk. A scorpion's sting causes immediate pain and burning around the sting site, followed by numbness or tingling. Severe cases usually appear only in small children and may include paralysis, spasms, or respiratory difficulties. First aid consists of monitoring the ABCs and treating the victim accordingly. It is also important to clean the sting site with soap and water or rubbing alcohol and then apply an ice pack over the wound. Seek medical attention.

Tick Removal

Most tick bites are harmless, though ticks can carry serious diseases (e.g., Lyme disease, Rocky Mountain spotted fever, Colorado tick fever.) Ticks should be removed as soon as possible. Because of its painless bite, a tick can remain embedded for days without the human victim ever knowing. An embedded tick in the hairy parts of the body (i.e., scalp, armpit, pubis) may go undetected and may be passed off as a dark mole.

First Aid

- Do *not* use the following popular methods of tick removal, which have proven useless:
    1. Petroleum jelly
    2. Fingernail polish
    3. Rubbing alcohol

Lyme Disease

Lyme Disease is the most common tick-borne disease, and its occurrence is fast-rising in almost all states. Lyme disease (named for the Connecticut town in which it was first discovered) starts out with flu-like symptoms, but can lead to arthritis and serious nerve and heart damage. Ticks carrying the disease often go undetected since they are difficult to see and are much smaller (head of a pin in size) than the common dog tick or wood tick.

Protection against ticks comes from taking these precautions:

1. Wear long-sleeved shirts and long pants (tucked into socks) whenever in wooded areas.

2. Use insect repellent containing DEET (diethyltolusmide) on clothes and exposed areas, especially arms and hands.

3. Check yourself for ticks or have someone do it for you after being in a potentially tick-infested area.

4. Immediately remove any embedded tick with tweezers.

5. Consult with a physician if any flu-like symptoms occur (chills, pain).

■ TICK REMOVAL ■

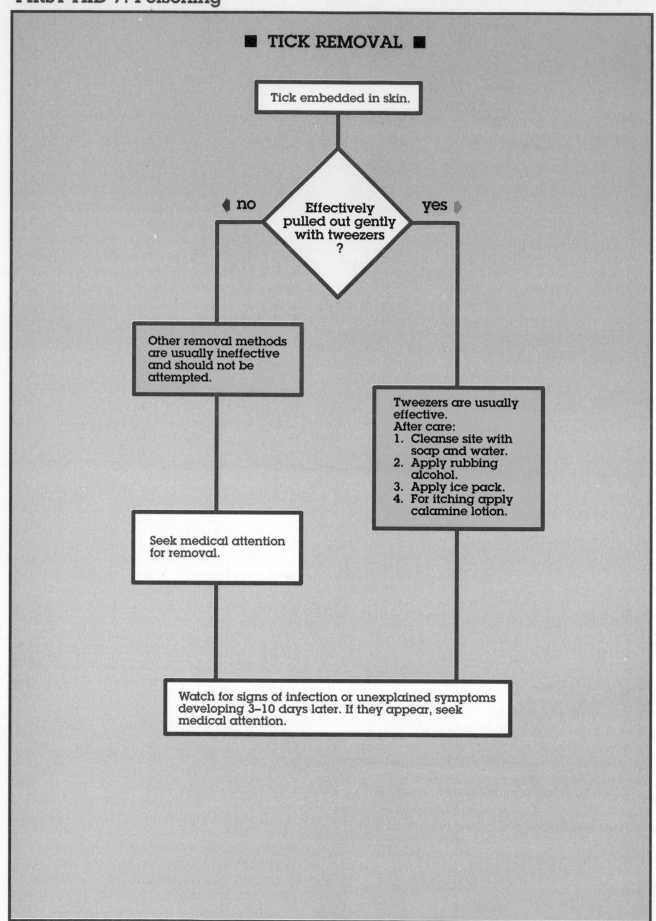

Tick embedded in skin.

Effectively pulled out gently with tweezers?

no

yes

Other removal methods are usually ineffective and should not be attempted.

Tweezers are usually effective.
After care:
1. Cleanse site with soap and water.
2. Apply rubbing alcohol.
3. Apply ice pack.
4. For itching apply calamine lotion.

Seek medical attention for removal.

Watch for signs of infection or unexplained symptoms developing 3–10 days later. If they appear, seek medical attention.

4. A hot match

■ Pull the tick off, employing the following methods:

1. Use tweezers, or if you have to use your fingers, protect your skin by using a paper towel or disposable tissue. Although few people ever encounter ticks infected with a disease, the person removing the tick may become infected by germs entering through breaks in the skin.

2. Grasp the tick as close to the skin surface as possible and pull away from the skin with a steady pressure or lift the tick slightly upward and pull parallel to the skin until the tick detaches. Do *not* twist or jerk the tick since this may result in incomplete removal.

3. Wash the bite site and your hands well with soap and water. Apply alcohol to further disinfect the area. Then apply a cold pack to reduce pain. Calamine lotion might aid in relieving any itching. Keep the area clean.

Watch for signs of infection or unexplained symptoms (e.g., severe headaches, fever, or rash) which may develop 3 to 10 days later. If these symptoms appear, seek medical attention immediately.

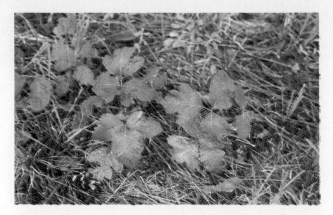

Poison oak

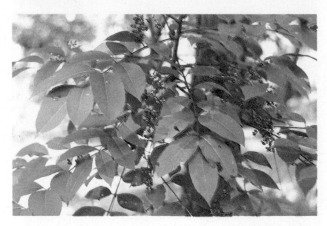

Poison sumac

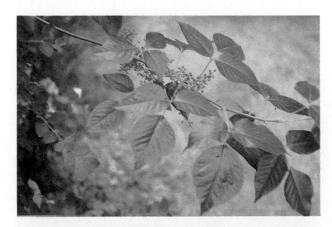

Poison ivy, found in all 48 contiguous U.S. states

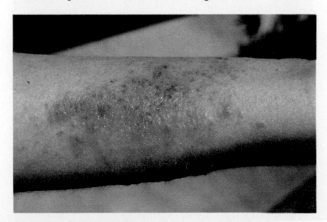

Poison ivy dermatitis

Poison Ivy, Oak, and Sumac

Poison ivy, oak, and sumac plants cause contact dermatitis or an allergic reaction in about 90 percent of all adults. Most people cannot recognize these plants. To find out whether or not a plant is poisonous upon contact, use the "black spot test." (*See* boxed information). Actually, more than 60 plants can cause an allergic reaction, but the three named above are by far the most common offenders.

Allergic people may come in contact with the juice of these plants from their clothes or shoes, from pet fur, or from smoke of burning plants. No one can develop the dermatitis by touching the fluid from blisters, since that fluid does not contain the oleoresin that comes from the juice of these poisonous plants.

Signs and Symptoms

■ *Mild.* Some itching
■ *Mild to moderate.* Itching and redness
■ *Moderate.* Itching, redness, and swelling
■ *Severe.* Itching, redness, swelling, and blisters

Severity is important but so is the amount of skin affected. The greater the skin involvement, the greater

■ POISON IVY ■

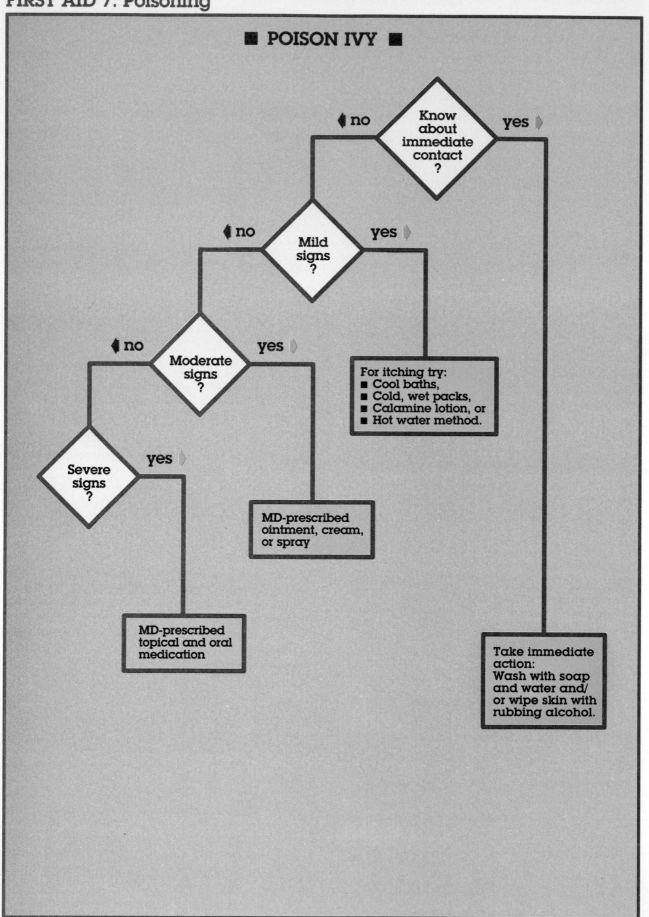

Know about immediate contact?

no ◄   yes ►

Mild signs?

no ◄   yes ►

Moderate signs?

no ◄   yes ►

Severe signs?

yes ►

For itching try:
■ Cool baths,
■ Cold, wet packs,
■ Calamine lotion, or
■ Hot water method.

MD-prescribed ointment, cream, or spray

MD-prescribed topical and oral medication

Take immediate action: Wash with soap and water and/ or wipe skin with rubbing alcohol.

the need for medical attention. A day or two is the usual time between contact and the onset of the above signs and symptoms.

First Aid

- Those knowing that they have contacted a poisonous plant should take immediate action (within 5 minutes). That action includes rinsing with plain water or using alcohol. Most victims do not know they have contacted a poisonous plant until the next day or later when the itching and rash begin.
- During the acute weeping and oozing stage, sodium bicarbonate (baking soda) solution should be used either as a soak, bath, or wet dressing for 30 minutes, three or four times a day. Greasy ointments should not be used during active oozing.
- Antihistamines appear to have no value either taken by mouth or in ointments and lotions. In fact, ointments and lotions could even cause their own allergic reactions on top of the poison plant eruption.
- For the various stages:

   1. *Mild.* Apply wet compresses and cool baths to help relieve itching. Calamine lotion or zinc oxide may also relieve itching. Topical over-the-counter medications are no more effective than these few simple procedures.

   2. *Mild to moderate.* Doctor-prescribed corticosteroids help. Over-the-counter (nonprescription) hydrocortisone creams, ointments and sprays in strengths of .5% or less offer little benefit.

   3. *Severe.* Doctor-prescribed oral corticosteriods (e.g., prednisone) may benefit victims affected most severely. Topical corticosteroid may also be applied. When using a topical cream, cover the affected area with a transparent plastic wrap and lightly bind with an elastic or self-adhering bandage.

Black Spot Test

Check a suspicious-looking plant to determine if it's poison ivy, oak, or sumac by grasping a leaf with a piece of paper and crushing it with a rock. The sap of poison ivy, oak, and sumac will turn dark brown in 10 minutes, and turn black in a day.

—*Dr. Jere Guin, University of Arkansas*

For severe itching, hot water—hot enough to redden the skin, but not burn it—may relieve itching. Heat releases histamine, the substance in the skin's cells that causes the intense itching. Therefore, a hot shower or bath causes intense itching as the histamine is released. This depletes the cells of histamine and the victim will then obtain up to eight hours of relief from itching.

Carbon Monoxide

Victims of carbon monoxide (CO) are often unaware of its presence. The gas is invisible, tasteless, odorless and nonirritating.

Carbon monoxide produces its toxicity due to several factors. CO becomes tightly bound to hemoglobin (red blood cells) that carries oxygen. With conscious victims it takes four to five hours with ordinary air (21% oxygen) or 30–40 minutes with 100% oxygen to reverse CO's effects. When CO levels in the air are high, the level of oxygen is probably low.

Signs and Symptoms

It is difficult to tell if a person is a victim of carbon monoxide poisoning. Sometimes, a complaint of having the "flu" is really a symptom of carbon monoxide poisoning.

- Headache
- Ringing in the ears (tinnitus)
- Angina (chest pain)
- Muscle weakness
- Nausea and vomiting
- Dizziness and visual changes (blurred or double vision)
- Unconsciousness
- Breathing and cardiac failure

First Aid

- Immediately remove the victim from the toxic environment and into fresh air. Give the victim 100% oxygen either in an EMS ambulance or at a hospital emergency department. This will improve oxygenation and it also disassociates the linkage between the carbon monoxide and the hemoglobin.
- For a conscious victim, seek medical attention involving a blood test to determine the level of carbon monoxide.
- For an unconscious victim, place him or her on one side with the head resting on an arm. Loosen tight clothing and maintain body heat.
- Give basic life support if needed.
- Even when only mild symptoms (e.g., headache, nausea) appear, seek medical attention if carbon monoxide poisoning suspected.

■ INHALED POISON ■

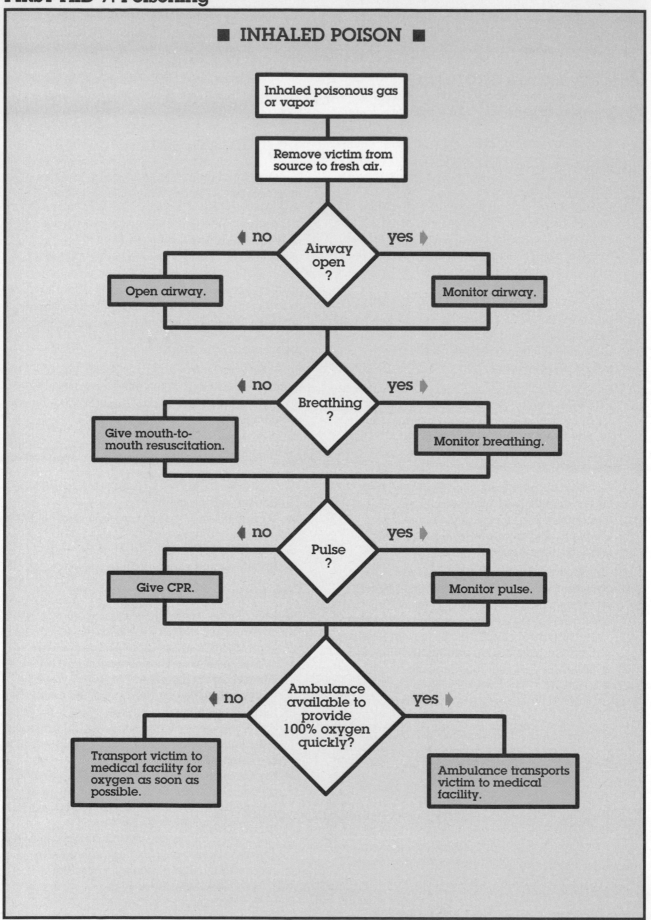

■ ACTIVITY 1 ■
Swallowed Poison

Check the appropriate question(s).

You suspect a 3-year-old boy has swallowed aspirin from an opened bottle. What information should you immediately attempt to find out?

1. ____ Did he eat any aspirin?
2. ____ How many tablets, if any, did he eat?
3. ____ If he ate any aspirin, how long has it been?

Mark each action yes (Y) or no (N).

If an elderly man reports he swallowed a substance that you know is poisonous, you should . . .

1. ____ Ask him how much he took, and when.
2. ____ Give him a glass of milk to drink.
3. ____ Telephone the poison control center and tell them what you know about the poisoning.

4. ____ Empty the victim's stomach before attempting to contact a medical authority.

Mark the following statements true (T) or false (F).

1. ____ Always induce vomiting with syrup of ipecac in a conscious person who has swallowed a poison.
2. ____ Give syrup of ipecac for poisoning only after receiving medical advice or when told to do so by a poison control center.
3. ____ Syrup of ipecac alone causes vomiting.
4. ____ Gagging or drinking warm salt water are as effective and safe as syrup of ipecac for inducing vomiting.

■ ACTIVITY 2 ■
Insect Stings

Mark each action yes (Y) or no (N).

Which are appropriate first aid measures for insect stings?

1. ____ Remove a stinger with tweezers or fingers.
2. ____ Wash the stung area with soap and water.
3. ____ Place a warm pack over the stung area.

4. ____ Immediately seek medical attention for the victim with prior reactions.
5. ____ For allergic reactions, use epinephrine from an emergency insect sting kit.

■ ACTIVITY 3 ■
Snakebites

Choose the best answer.

Which should you do for a venomous snakebite?

1. ____ **A.** Cool the bite site with ice.
    B. Avoid using cold on the bite site.
2. ____ **A.** Avoid cutting through any snakebite wound.
    B. Cut through the bite wound if you are several hours from a medical facility.

3. ____ **A.** First aiders can give antivenin.
    B. Only qualified medical personnel should give antivenin.
4. ____ **A.** Apply a tourniquet.
    B. Apply suction with the Extractor™.
5. ____ **A.** If possible, identify the snake and its size.
    B. Information about the snake isn't usually needed.

■ ACTIVITY 4 ■
Spider Bites and Scorpion Stings

Mark each action yes (Y) or no (N).

Which of the following first aid procedures are appropriate for spider bites and scorpion stings?

1. _____ Apply a cold or ice pack over the bite site.
2. _____ Seek medical attention immediately.
3. _____ Apply a constriction band 2–4 inches above the bite.
4. _____ Capture the spider or have a definite identification.
5. _____ Apply calamine lotion to relieve pain.
6. _____ Wash area with soap and water or rubbing alcohol.

■ ACTIVITY 5 ■
Tick Removal

Check (✓) the best answers.

Choose the methods that are most likely to be successful in removing an embedded tick.

1. _____ Apply a substance (e.g., oil or grease) to smother the tick, causing it to disengage its head.
2. _____ Apply fingernail polish and allow it to harden. Peel the polish off and the tick will come with it.
3. _____ Apply heat by holding a heated needle or a blown-out, glowing match head to the tick.
4. _____ Pull the embedded tick out with tweezers.
5. _____ Pry a tick out with a needle.
6. _____ Put some gasoline or rubbing alcohol on a cotton ball and tape it loosely over the tick for 15 minutes.
7. _____ Apply an ice cube over the tick.

■ ACTIVITY 6 ■
Poison Ivy, Oak, and Sumac

Check the appropriate action(s).

Which of the following may be useful in alleviating itching caused by poison ivy, oak, or sumac?

1. _____ Apply rubbing alcohol to the rash and all affected areas.
2. _____ Apply calamine lotion to the affected areas.
3. _____ Take an antihistamine.
4. _____ Apply hot water (not hot enough to burn) even though it will produce intense itching initially.
5. _____ Get a physician's prescription for a corticosteroid.
6. _____ Wash the affected areas with water immediately after contact with the plant.

■ ACTIVITY 7 ■
Carbon Monoxide Poisoning

Mark the statement true (T) or false (F).

1. _____ Carbon monoxide (CO) from automobiles is easily detected by its odor.
2. _____ Headache characterizes carbon monoxide poisoning.
3. _____ Carbon monoxide victims need pure oxygen as quickly as possible.
4. _____ Check with a physician whenever carbon monoxide poisoning is suspected.
5. _____ Carbon monoxide poisoning symptoms can be confused with those of viral infections (flu).

8

Burns

■ Heat Burns ■ Chemical Burns ■
■ Electrical Burns ■

Heat Burns

More than two million burn injuries each year require medical attention or restriction of activity. Of these, about one-third are treated at hospital emergency departments. More than 6,000 persons die annually from injuries caused by burns.

The skin is sensitive to heat. Skin damage usually does not occur below 111°F. Temperatures between 111° and 123° cause significant tissue damage. Temperatures above 123° destroy skin within a brief moment.

Assessing a Burn

Assess a burn after any breathing or bleeding problems have been treated.

Controversy about whether or not first aiders should perform a burn assessment exists. Some authorities agree that it may be difficult to accurately determine the percentage and depth of a burn during the initial stages. They contend that such estimates are better done after waiting several days when the tissues become more clearly defined. On the other hand, many other experts contend that while that may be true, an attempt should be made since it is important to have an assessment for proper first aid. Therefore, a rapid but complete assessment is recommended.

How large is the burn?

The extent of a burn is expressed as a percentage of the total body surface. The familiar "Rule of Nines" defines a hand and arm as 9% of the body surface. Each leg counts as 18% of the body surface. The front and back torso are each valued at 18% with the genital area at 1%. The victim's hand size is about 1% and this surface area can be used for calculating most burns.

The Rule of Nines is accurate for adults, but it does not make allowances for the different proportions of a child. In small children the head accounts for 18% and each leg 14%. Accordingly, the Rule of Nines is modified.

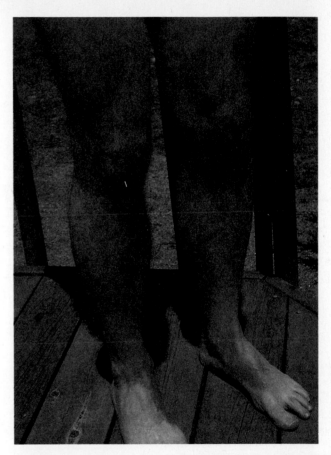

First-degree burn—sunburned legs

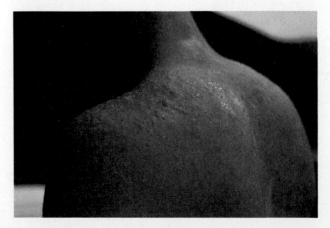

Second-degree burn—blistered shoulders

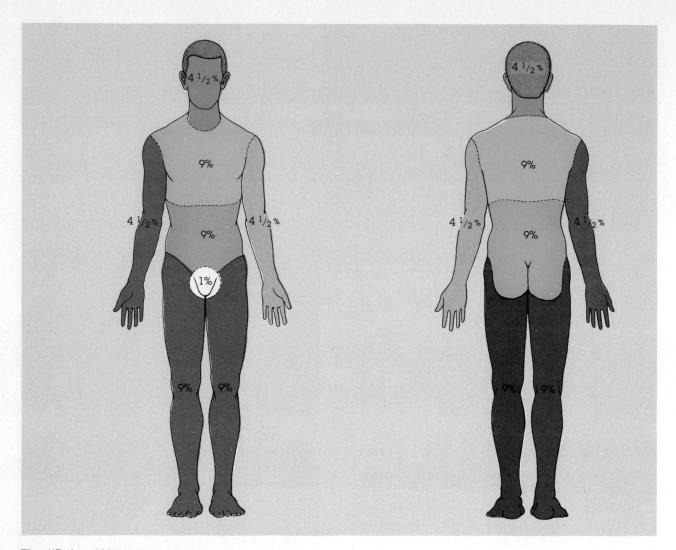

The "Rule of Nines"

How deep is the burn?

First-degree burns (superficial). These burns affect the skin's outer layer. Characteristics include redness, mild swelling, tenderness, and pain.

Second-degree burns (partial-thickness). These burns extend through the entire outer skin layer and into the inner skin layer. Blister formation, swelling, weeping of fluids, and severe pain characterize second-degree burns. Intact blisters maintain a sterile waterproof covering of the wound. Once a blister breaks, a weeping wound results.

Third-degree burns (full-thickness). These severe burns extend through all the skin layers and into the underlying fat, muscle, and bone. Discoloration (charred, white, or cherry red) and a leathery, parchmentlike, dry appearance indicate this degree of burn. Pain is absent because the nerve endings have been destroyed. Any pain found with this burn results from accompanying burns of lesser degrees (first- and second-degree). Proper healing requires skin grafting.

What parts of the body are burned?

Areas of most importance are the face (especially the eyelids), the hands, the feet, and the genitals. Respiratory tract burns are especially serious if associated with inhalation of fumes or heat.

How old is the burned victim?

A burn is considered more serious in an infant and in an elderly person (over 65) than in other victims.

Does the victim have any injuries or medical problems?

Burns can aggravate diabetes, heart disease, and lung disease, as well as other medical problems.

With this information and reference to Table 8.1, the burn's severity can be determined as minor, moderate, or major (critical).

General First Aid

1. Put out the fire. Clothing fires should be immediately extinguished by having the victim "drop and roll," or by wrapping the victim in a blanket.

TABLE 8–1 Burn Severity

Burn classification	Characteristics	
Minor burn	first-degree burn	
	second-degree burn	<15% BSA adults
	second-degree burn	<5% BSA in children/elderly persons
	third-degree burn	<2% BSA
Moderate burn	second-degree burn	15%–25% BSA in adults
	second-degree burn	10%–20% BSA in children/elderly persons
	third-degree burn	<10% BSA
Critical burn	second-degree burn	>25% BSA in adults
	second-degree burn	>20% BSA in children/elderly persons
	third-degree burn	>10% BSA
		Burns of hands, face, eyes, feet, or perineum
		Most victims with inhalation injury, electrical injury, major trauma, or significant preexisting diseases

BSA = Body surface area
Source: Adapted with permission from the American Burn Association categorization.

2. Move the victim away from a burning area to avoid further injury.

3. Remove smoldering clothing or soak it with cold water.

4. Do *not* try to remove clothing that is stuck to the skin—cut around the clothing and do *not* pull on it because pulling will damage the skin. Remove jewelry, such as rings, from the burned area as soon as possible, since they retain heat, and swelling could make it difficult to remove them later.

5. Immerse the burned area in cold water for about 10 minutes. This is effective only in the 30–45 minutes immediately after injury. Do *not* apply cold on large burned areas (i.e., greater than 20%).

6. Other types of injuries take first aid priority over a burn (except chemical burns). Examine burned victims, except chemically burned victims, as though the burn injury did not exist.

7. Do *not* break any blisters.

8. Cover the burn with a dry sterile gauze dressing. Large areas may require a clean cloth (e.g., a pillowcase, towel, or sheet).

Do *not* place a moist dressing over a burn since it dries out quickly and adheres to the burn as it dries. Also, moist dressings over a large area can induce hypothermia. Wet compresses should be limited to initially cooling a burn; they do not serve as a dressing.

Do *not* use an occlusive dressing (its only advantage is that it does not stick to the burn) since it prevents the loss of moisture and is a good place for bacteria to grow. This can lead to infection.

9. Do *not* put any type of ointment, grease, lotion, butter, antiseptic, or home remedies on burned skin. These methods are unsterile and may lead to infection. Moreover, they can seal in the heat, resulting in further damage. Often, a physician will have to scrape them off in order to give proper treatment. This is a very painful experience for the victim.

10. Monitor breathing and watch for respiratory distress.

11. Treat the victim for shock by elevating the legs 8 to 12 inches and keeping him or her warm.

12. Burn victims are susceptible to hypothermia because they lose large amounts of heat and water through burned tissue. Keep the victim warm.

First-degree burns

Apply cold water until the pain stops. Cold water from most home faucets is usually cold enough. Ice is not needed.

Fast cooling aids healing. Recommended times for cold applications vary from 10 minutes to 30 minutes, while some suggest its application until the pain does not recur after cold is discontinued. Frostbite can happen when cold is misused. Do *not* apply directly to the burned area; protect the skin by wrapping the ice in a cloth.

Second-degree burns (small area)

Apply cold water until the pain stops.

Do *not* break any blisters. They provide a protective covering against bacteria.

Third-degree and large second-degree burns

1. Check immediately for an open airway, breathing, and circulation. Give mouth-to-mouth resuscitation and CPR if necessary.

TABLE 8-2 First Aid for Burns

Burn	Do	Don't
First-degree (redness, mild swelling, and pain)	Apply cold water and/or dry sterile dressing.	Apply butter, oleomargarine, etc.
Second-degree (deeper; blisters develop)	Immerse in cold water, blot dry with sterile cloth for protection. Treat for shock. Obtain medical attention if severe.	Break blisters. Remove shreds of tissue. Use antiseptic preparation, ointment spray, or home remedy on severe burn.
Third-degree (deeper destruction, skin layers destroyed)	Cover with sterile cloth to protect. Treat for shock. Watch for breathing difficulty. Obtain medical attention quickly.	Remove charred clothing that is stuck to burn. Apply ice. Use home medication.
Chemical Burn	Remove by flushing with large quantities of water for at least 15 minutes. Remove surrounding clothing. Obtain medical attention.	Neutralize

Source: U.S. Coast Guard.

Later Burn Care

Follow a physician's recommendations about burn care, if there are any (many burns are never seen by a doctor). The following suggestions apply to such situations:

1. Wash hands thoroughly before changing any dressing.

2. Leave unbroken blisters intact.

3. Change dressings two times a day unless told otherwise by a physician.

4. Change a dressing by:
   a. Removing old dressings. If a dressing sticks, soak it off with cool, clean water.
   b. Cleanse area gently with mild soap and water.
   c. Pat area dry with clean cloth.
   d. Apply a thin layer of antibacterial cream to the burn.
   e. Apply sterile dressings.

5. Watch for signs of infection. Call a physician if any of these appear:
   a. Increased redness, pain, tenderness, swelling, or red streaks near burn
   b. Pus
   c. Elevated temperature (fever)

6. Keep the area and dressing as clean and dry as possible.

7. Elevate the burned area, if possible, for the first 24 hours.

8. Give a pain medication if necessary.

2. Treat for shock by elevating the legs 8 to 12 inches and keeping the victim warm.

3. Do *not* open any blisters or remove pieces of tissue from the burned skin.

4. Do *not* apply cold to a third-degree or large second-degree burn. The burned victim's body heat must be conserved since hypothermia may be induced.

5. Apply sterile dressings or, if they are not available, clean cloths.

6. Elevate burned arms or legs to reduce swelling and pain.

Chemical Burns

At least 25,000 products found in industry, agriculture, and the home can burn and cause tissue damage. A chemical continues to cause damage until it is inactivated by the tissue, is neutralized, or is diluted with water. The "burning" process may continue for long periods of time after initial contact. Alkali burns are more serious than acid burns because they penetrate deeper and remain active longer.

Toxicology training is not needed to treat all of the common chemical burns because first aid is the same for all except a few special burns for which something has to be added to neutralize the chemical.

First Aid

- Wash with large quantities of water all liquid acids, alkalis, and caustic agents. In acid and

■ HEAT BURNS ■

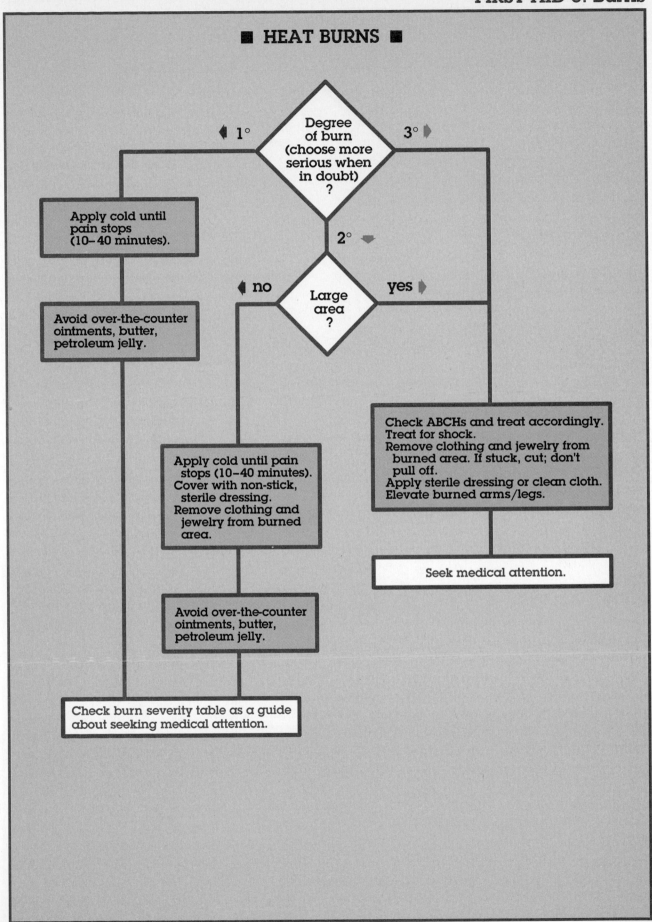

Degree of burn (choose more serious when in doubt)?

◀ 1°   3° ▶

2° ▶

1°:
Apply cold until pain stops (10–40 minutes).

Avoid over-the-counter ointments, butter, petroleum jelly.

Check burn severity table as a guide about seeking medical attention.

Large area?

◀ no   yes ▶

no:
Apply cold until pain stops (10–40 minutes). Cover with non-stick, sterile dressing. Remove clothing and jewelry from burned area.

Avoid over-the-counter ointments, butter, petroleum jelly.

yes:
Check ABCHs and treat accordingly. Treat for shock. Remove clothing and jewelry from burned area. If stuck, cut; don't pull off. Apply sterile dressing or clean cloth. Elevate burned arms/legs.

Seek medical attention.

■ CHEMICAL BURNS ■

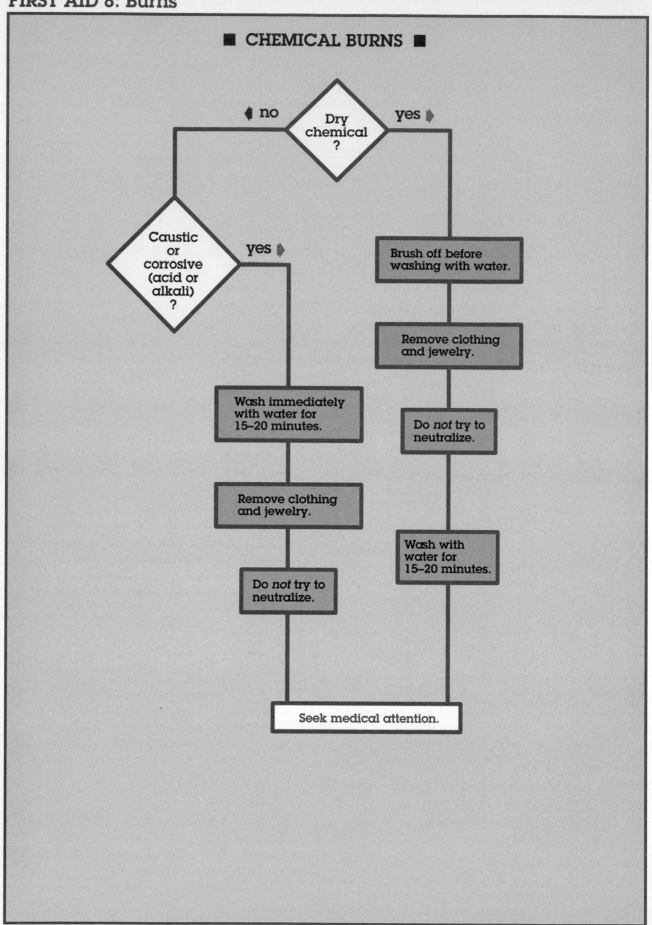

Dry chemical?

no ◀   **yes** ▶

Caustic or corrosive (acid or alkali)?

yes ▶

Brush off before washing with water.

Remove clothing and jewelry.

Wash immediately with water for 15–20 minutes.

Do *not* try to neutralize.

Remove clothing and jewelry.

Wash with water for 15–20 minutes.

Do *not* try to neutralize.

Seek medical attention.

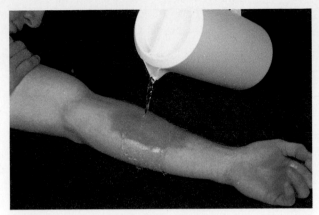
Washing/flooding chemical burns

alkali burns, damage is practically set within three minutes after the victim comes in contact with the chemical, so flushing the victim's burns with water in the first minutes after contact substantially reduces the damage.

■ Removing contaminated clothing takes any absorbed chemicals away from the skin. Do this while washing the victim.

■ Do *not* apply water under any type of pressure because pressure drives the chemical deeper into the tissue. Use a faucet or hose under low pressure and wash with a gentle flow for long periods of time—even for one or more hours.

■ Brush off a dry or solid chemical substance (e.g., lime) before flushing with water. Water activates a dry chemical and will cause more damage to the skin than when it is dry.

■ Do *not* attempt to neutralize a chemical because heat may be produced, resulting in more damage. Some product label directions for neutralizing may be wrong. Save the container or label for the name of the chemical.

■ Call a poison control center to find out other steps you can take. Additional treatments would be the same as for any heat burn of the same extent and depth.

Electrical Burns

Electrical injuries are devastating. Even with just a mild shock, a victim can suffer serious internal injuries. A current of 1,000 volts or more is considered high voltage, but even the 110 volts of household current can be deadly.

High voltage electrical currents passing through the body may disrupt the normal heart rhythm, cause cardiac arrest, burns, and other injuries.

When someone is electrocuted, electricity enters the body at the point of contact and travels along the path of least resistance (nerves and blood vessels). The current travels rapidly, generating heat and causing destruction. Usually, the electricity exits where the body is touching a surface or is in contact with a ground (e.g., a metal object). Sometimes, a victim may have more than one exit site.

Contact with Power Line (Outside Situations)

If electrocution comes from contact with a downed power line, the power must be turned off before a rescuer approaches anyone who may be in contact with the wire.

If the victim is in a car with a power line fallen across it, tell him or her to stay in the car until the power can be shut off. The only exception to this rule is when fire threatens the car. In this case, tell the victim to jump out of the car without making contact with the car or wire.

If you approach a victim and you feel a tingling sensation in your legs and lower body, stop. This sensation signals you are on energized ground and that an electrical current is entering through one foot, passing through your lower body, and leaving through the other foot. If this happens, raise a foot off the ground, turn around and hop to a safe place.

If you can safely reach the victim, do *not* attempt to move any wires with wood poles, tools with wood handles, or objects with a high moisture content. Do *not* attempt to move downed wires at all unless you are trained and equipped with tools able to handle the high voltage.

Wait until the power company can cut the wires or disconnect them. Prevent bystanders from entering the danger area.

Contact Inside Buildings

Most electrical burns inside occur from faulty electrical equipment or careless use of electrical appliances. Turn off the electricity at the circuit breaker, fuse box, outside switch box, or unplug the appliance if the plug is undamaged. Do *not* touch the appliance or the victim until the current is off.

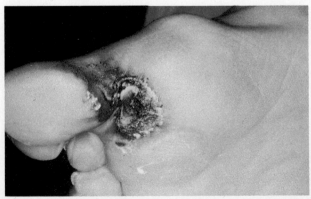
Electrical burn—toe

■ ELECTRICAL INJURIES ■

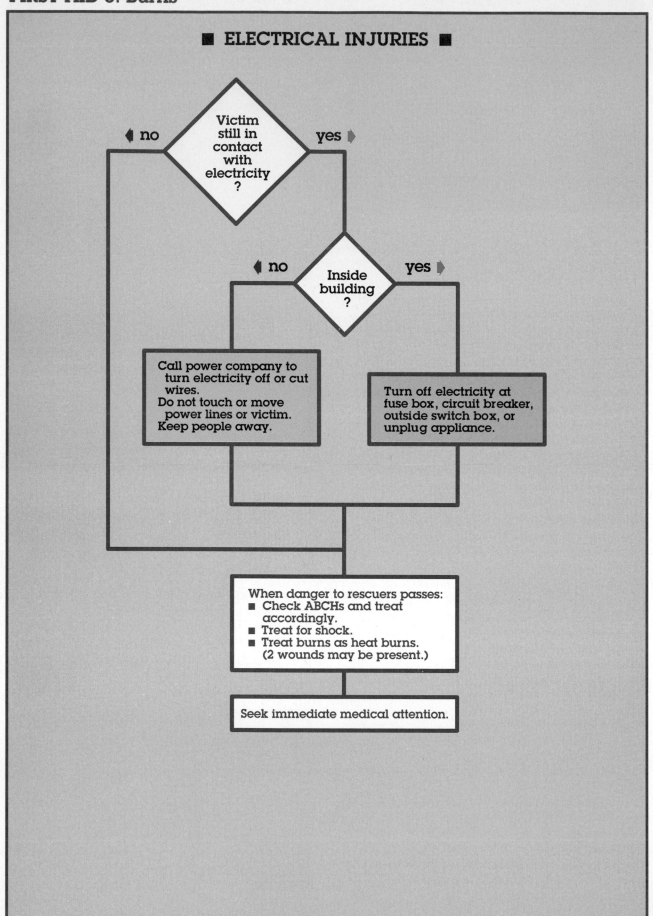

Victim still in contact with electricity ?

◀ no   yes ▶

Inside building ?

◀ no   yes ▶

Call power company to turn electricity off or cut wires.
Do not touch or move power lines or victim.
Keep people away.

Turn off electricity at fuse box, circuit breaker, outside switch box, or unplug appliance.

When danger to rescuers passes:
■ Check ABCHs and treat accordingly.
■ Treat for shock.
■ Treat burns as heat burns. (2 wounds may be present.)

Seek immediate medical attention.

First Aid

Once the danger to rescuers has passed, first aid can begin.

- Check the ABCs—airway, breathing, and circulation and treat accordingly.
- Check for burns and treat for shock by elevating the legs 8 to 12 inches and keeping the victim warm. Most electrical burns are third-degree burns, so cover them with a sterile dressing and elevate the part.

Electrical current flows quickly into the body's tissues, then exits. The surface injuries of the skin involve small surface areas (entrance and exit points); the major damage occurs deep under the skin. Any major electrical incident must be handled as if this were the case.

All victims of electrical shock should receive immediate medical attention.

Lightning Strikes

The main concern with a lightning injury is the possibility of respiratory or cardiac arrest. Many times, lightning will not strike a victim directly. Instead, it bounces off a nearby structure, then hits the victim.

First Aid

First aiders must start aggressive, vigorous resuscitation for victims of cardiac arrest. First aid begins with the ABCs. Open the airway by using the jaw thrust

Lightning-Related deaths, 1959–1987

States where deaths attributed to lightning occur most frequently (in descending order):

1. Florida
2. North Carolina
3. Texas
4. Tennessee
5. New York
6. Maryland
7. Louisiana
8. Arkansas
9. Ohio
10. Pennsylvania

Places where people are killed by lightning most often (with percent of deaths):

In open fields	27%
Under trees	17%
On or near water	12%
Near tractors/ heavy equipment	6%
On golf courses	4%
At telephones	1%
Other	33%

—National Oceanic and Atmospheric Administration

Avoiding Being Struck by Lightning

The first line of defense is to know when and where you can be hit by lightning. Some parts of the day are riskier than others. According to studies, about 70% of lightning injuries and deaths occur in the afternoon, 20% between 6:00 P.M. and midnight, 10% between 7 A.M. and noon, and fewer than 1% from midnight to 6:00 A.M. Lightning is also far more common from May through September than in other months.

Armed with these facts, protect yourself when a thunderstorm threatens. Get inside a home or large building, or inside an all-metal (not convertible) vehicle. Inside a home, avoid using the telephone, except for emergencies. If you are outside, with no time to reach a safe building or an automobile, follow these rules:

- Do not stand underneath a natural lightning rod such as a tall, isolated tree in an open area.
- Avoid projecting above the surrounding landscape, as you would do if you were standing on a hilltop, in an open field, on the beach, or fishing from a small boat.
- Get out of and away from open water.
- Get away from tractors and other metal farm equipment.
- Get off and away from motorcycles, scooters, golf carts, and bicycles. Put down golf clubs.
- Stay away from wire fences, clotheslines, metal pipes, rails, and other metallic parts which could carry lightning to you from some distance away.
- Avoid standing in small, isolated sheds or other small structures in open areas.
- In a forest, seek shelter in a low area under a thick growth of small trees. In open areas, go to a low place such as a ravine or valley. Be alert for flash floods.
- If you're hopelessly isolated in a level field or prairie and you feel your hair stand on end—indicating lightning is about to strike—drop to your knees and bend forward, putting your hands on your knees. *Do not* lie flat on the ground. This will ensure that as small an area as possible is touching the ground and will minimize the danger of your body acting as a conductor.

—National Oceanic and Atmospheric Administration

The only man in the world to be struck by lightning 7 times is former Shenandoah Park Ranger Roy C. Sullivan. His attraction for lightning began in 1942 (lost big toenail) and was resumed in July 1969 (lost eyebrows), in July 1970 (left shoulder seared), on April 16, 1972 (hair set on fire) and, finally, he hoped, on August 7, 1973: as he was driving along a bolt came out of a small, low-lying cloud, hit him on the head through his hat, set his hair on fire again, knocked him 10 feet out of his car, went through both legs, and knocked his left shoe off. He had to pour a pail of water over his head to cool off. Then, on June 5, 1976, he was struck again for the sixth time, his ankle injured. When he was struck for the *seventh* time on June 25, 1977, while fishing, he was sent to Waynesboro Hospital with chest and stomach burns. In September 1983, reportedly rejected in love, he died of a self-inflicted gunshot wound.

—*Guinness Book of World Records*

method in order to avoid neck hyperextension, which may result in a neck spine injury.

If the victim is in cardiac arrest, start CPR. Persistent first aid is crucial for these victims. Treat for shock. Since spinal cord injuries can occur with lightning strikes, precautions should be taken for immobilizing the spine.

If more than one victim has been struck by lightning at the same time, give the highest priority to those in cardiac arrest.

Lightning-struck victims are not charged with electricity and do not represent a hazard to the first aider.

■ ACTIVITY 1 ■
Heat Burns

Choose the best answer.

1. ____ What should you do first to ease the pain from a burn?
   A. Hold the injured part in a sink filled with warm water.
   B. Cover the burned area with a clean dressing.
   C. Cover the burn with petroleum jelly or any over-the-counter burn ointment.
   D. Place the injured part in a sink filled with running cold water.

2. ____ How could you lessen pain while seeking medical assistance for a burned victim?
   A. Soak burned area in warm water.
   B. Cover small burned areas with cool wet cloths.
   C. Pinch the areas.
   D. Immerse in cold saltwater.

3. ____ The type of burn characterized by reddening, blisters and deep, intense pain is called a:
   A. First-degree burn
   B. Second-degree burn
   C. Third-degree burn

4. ____ Which type of burn is characterized by little or no pain and skin that is usually charred black or has areas that are dry and white?
   A. First-degree burn
   B. Second-degree burn
   C. Third-degree burn

5. ____ Using the "Rule of Nines," what percentage of an adult's body is involved if one entire arm and the front of one leg are burned?
   A. 9%
   B. 18%
   C. 27%
   D. 36%

6. ____ Which body areas are especially sensitive to being burned?
   A. Face
   B. Hands
   C. Feet
   D. All of the above

7. ____ A victim's hand size represents what percentage of the body?
   A. 1%
   B. 5%
   C. 10%

Mark each action yes (Y) or no (N).

When giving first aid for a burn, you should

1. ____ Apply petroleum jelly on the burn.
2. ____ Pull off a piece of clothing that is stuck to a burn.
3. ____ Apply a clean dressing and secure it in place.
4. ____ Blow on a burned area to cool it.
5. ____ Use your fingers to remove pieces of burned skin.
6. ____ Open blisters before applying a dressing.
7. ____ Apply cool water to the burn.

■ ACTIVITY 2 ■
Chemical Burns

Choose the best answer.

1. ____ First aid is the same for all types of chemical burns *except* a few special chemicals which need to be:
   A. neutralized
   B. treated without oxygen
   C. analyzed prior to treatment
   D. disinfected

2. ____ All acids, alkalies, and caustic agents are best treated by:
   A. neutralizing the chemicals
   B. applying petroleum products to the burn
   C. washing with large quantites of water
   D. wrapping the area to keep out oxygen

3. ____ When washing chemicals from the body, it is best if the water is:
A. applied to the area under high pressure
B. applied to the area under low pressure
C. considerably warmer than normal body temperature
D. kept in a large basin into which the part affected is submerged

4. ____ Which type of chemical substance may be activated if flushed with water?
A. dry chemicals
B. petroleum products
C. topical medications
D. fluid or wet chemicals

5. ____ Do not attempt to neutralize a chemical because the neutralization process may result in further damage due to:
A. mechanical irritation
B. the electricity produced
C. heat production
D. radiation effects

6. ____ What is the *first* step in caring for dry chemicals spilled on the skin?
A. Read the chemical container's label as to proper procedures.
B. Flush with water.
C. Brush off the substance before flushing with water.
D. Cover the area with sterile gauze.

■ ACTIVITY 3 ■
Electrical Burns

Choose the best answer.

1. ____ Household electricity, though damaging, is not deadly.
A. Yes
B. No

2. ____ When someone is electrocuted, how many burn wounds usually occur?
A. one
B. two
C. three or more

3. ____ If a victim is stranded in a car with a power line fallen across it, in most cases the victim should:
A. stay in the car
B. climb out of the car's window
C. jump from the car's window
D. exit through the door

4. ____ If you ever feel a tingling sensation in your legs when near a down electrical wire, you should:
A. raise a foot off the ground and hop to a safe place
B. continue walking through the area
C. run through the area
D. be concerned since the tingling indicates low voltage.

5. ____ If near a victim who is paralyzed by electrical current, you should:
A. try to move any wires with wood poles or handles
B. try to pull the victim from any wires
C. use wood poles or handles to try to pull the victim from any wires
D. wait until the power company can cut the wires or disconnect them

6. ____ Where does electricity produce the most damaging burns?
A. on the skin
B. deep under the skin

7. ____ First aid for a victim of electrical shock may include:
A. CPR
B. burn treatment
C. shock treatment
D. all of the above

9

Cold- and Heat-Related Emergencies

■ Frostbite ■ Hypothermia ■ Heat Stroke ■ Heat Exhaustion ■
■ Heat Cramps ■ Heat Syncope ■

Frostbite*

Frostbite occurs when temperatures drop below freezing. Tissue is damaged in two ways: (1) actual tissue freezing, which results in the formation of ice crystals between the tissue cells; the ice crystals enlarge by extracting water from the cells. and (2) the obstruction of blood supply to the tissues; this causes "sludged" blood clots, which prevent blood from flowing to the tissues. The second way injures more than the freezing does.

Frostbite mainly affects the feet, hands, ears, and nose. These areas do not contain large heat-producing muscles and are some distance from the heat generation sources. Moreover, when the body conserves heat, the blood supply diminishes in these areas first. The most severe consequences of frostbite are gangrene and amputation. Some people are more prone to frostbite than others. Victims may also suffer from hypothermia.

Frostnip happens after long cold exposure but is not a serious problem. The condition is not usually painful. The skin becomes white or pale. First aid for frostnip consists of gently warming the affected area. This can be done with bare hands or by blowing warm air on the area.

Signs and Symptoms (Classified by Thawing)

Types Based on the Pre-Thaw Stage

Superficial

- Skin color is white or grayish-yellow
- Pain may occur early and later subside
- Affected part may feel only very cold and numb. There may be a tingling, stinging, or aching sensation.
- Skin surface will feel hard or crusty and underlying tissue soft when depressed gently and firmly.

Source: Based on National Ski Patrol protocols; adapted with permission.

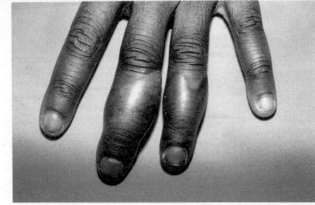

Frostbitten fingers, 6 hours after rewarming in 108°F water

Deep

- Affected part feels hard, solid, and cannot be depressed.
- Blisters appear in 12 to 36 hours.
- Affected part is cold with pale, waxy skin.
- A painfully cold part suddenly stops hurting.

Types Based on the Post-Thaw Stage

After a part has thawed, frostbite can be categorized into degrees similar to the classification of burns. First-degree frostbite is superficial, while the other three are degrees of deep frostbite.

- ***First-degree frostbite.*** Affected part is warm, swollen, and tender.
- ***Second-degree frostbite.*** Blisters form within minutes to hours after thawing and enlarge over several days.
- ***Third-degree frostbite.*** Blisters are small, contain reddish-blue or purplish fluid. Surrounding skin may have a red or blue color and may not blanch when pressure is applied.
- ***Fourth-degree frostbite.*** No blisters or swelling occurs. The part remains numb, cold, white-to-dark-purple in color.

First Aid

All frostbite injuries follow the same first aid treatment. Seek medical attention immediately. *Rewarming of frostbitten parts seldom takes place outside of a medi-*

■ FROSTBITE ■

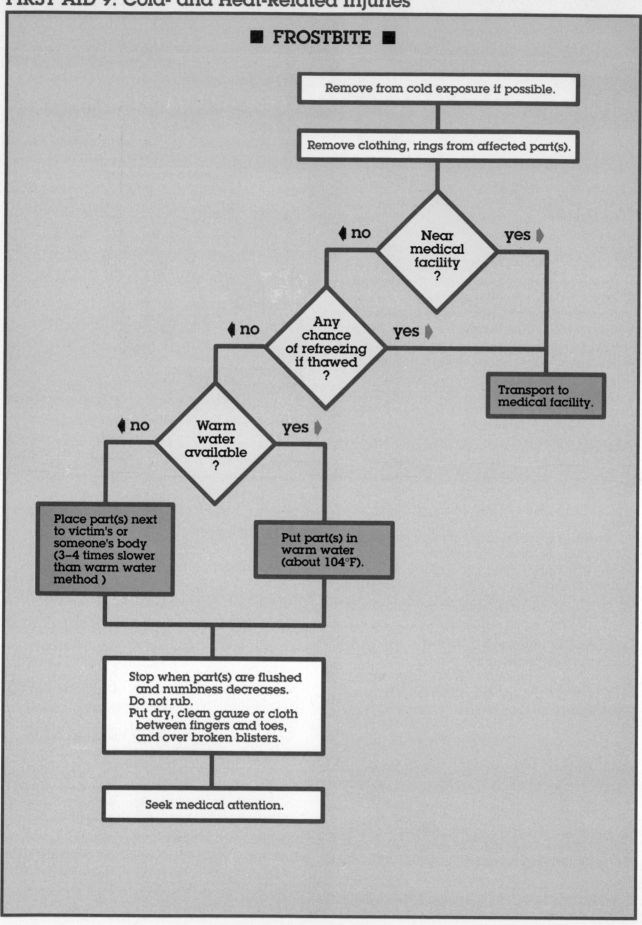

Remove from cold exposure if possible.

Remove clothing, rings from affected part(s).

Near medical facility?
— no
— yes

Any chance of refreezing if thawed?
— no
— yes

Warm water available?
— no
— yes

Transport to medical facility.

Place part(s) next to victim's or someone's body (3–4 times slower than warm water method)

Put part(s) in warm water (about 104°F).

Stop when part(s) are flushed and numbness decreases.
Do not rub.
Put dry, clean gauze or cloth between fingers and toes, and over broken blisters.

Seek medical attention.

cal facility because such facilities are usually nearby. However, if in a remote situation, the *wet, rapid rewarming method* may be used and is preferred to slow rewarming since the latter is associated with greater tissue damage.

Rapid Rewarming

- Do *not* attempt rewarming if a medical facility is nearby or if there is any chance that the part may refreeze.
- Remove any clothing or constricting items that could impair blood circulation (e.g., rings).
- Put the frostbitten part(s) in warm (not hot) water. Measure the water temperature with a thermometer. The water temperature should be 102–106°F. If you do not have a thermometer, test the water by pouring some water over the inside of your arm. Maintain the water temperature by adding warm water as needed.
- Warming usually takes 20 to 40 minutes and should be continued until the tissues are soft and pliable.
- For ear or facial injuries, apply warm moist cloths and change them frequently.
- To help control pain during the rewarming process, aspirin or ibuprofen may be given.

Post-Care

- Treat victim as a "stretcher" case.
- Maintain total body warmth.
- Protect injured part(s) from direct contact with clothing, bedding, etc.
- Leave any blisters intact.
- Place dry, sterile gauze between toes and fingers to absorb moisture and avoid having them stick together.
- Slightly elevate the affected part to reduce pain and swelling.
- Keep both the victim and affected part as warm as possible without overheating.

Cautions

- Do *not* allow the victim to walk on frostbitten toes or feet, especially after rewarming.
- Do *not* use water hotter than 106°F since burns can result.
- Do *not* allow the frostbitten part to freeze again since this can cause greater damage.
- Do *not* break any blisters that may have formed.
- Do *not* rub the part, even with snow.
- Do *not* rewarm the part with a heating pad, hot-water bottle, sunlamp, stove, radiator, exhaust pipe, or over a fire since this produces excessive temperatures and cannot be controlled, thus resulting in burns.
- Do *not* allow the victim to drink alcoholic beverages because they dilate blood vessels and cause a loss of body heat.
- Do *not* allow the victim to smoke since smoking constricts blood vessels, thus impairing circulation.
- Do *not* allow the thawed part to refreeze since ice crystals formed will be larger and more damaging.
- Unless circumstances justify its use (i.e., lack of water or fuel to warm water), do *not* use the "dry, rapid rewarming" technique (putting victim's hands in armpits) since it takes three to four times longer than the wet method to thaw frozen tissue and slow rewarming results in greater tissue damage than rapid rewarming.

How Cold Is It?

In addition to coldness, two other factors account for body heat loss: moisture and wind. Moisture—whether from rain, snow, or perspiration—speeds the conduction of heat away from the body.

Wind causes sizable amounts of body heat loss. If the thermometer reads 20°F and the wind speed is 20 mph, the exposure is comparable to −10°F. This is called the wind-chill factor. A rough measure of wind speed is: If you feel the wind on your face, the speed is about 10 mph; if small branches move or dust or snow is raised, 20 mph; if large branches are moving, 30 mph; and if a whole tree bends, about 40 mph.

Determine the wind-chill factor by:

1. Estimating the wind speed by checking for the signs described above.

2. Looking at a thermometer reading (in Fahrenheit degrees) outdoors.

3. Determining the wind-chill factor by matching the estimated wind speed with the actual thermometer reading in the "Wind-Chill Factor" table.

Hypothermia*

Hypothermia results from a cooling of the body's core temperature. Hypothermia can occur at temperatures above freezing as well as below it. The victim may suffer frostbite as well, if the body loses more heat than it produces. If the body temperature falls to 80°F, most people die. Hypothermia does not result from outdoor exposure alone. It is also caused by cool indoor temperatures.

Types of Exposure

1. *Acute exposure* occurs when the victim loses body heat very rapidly, usually in water immersion. Acute exposure is considered to be six hours or less in duration.

Source: Based on National Ski Patrol protocols; adapted with permission.

2. *Subacute exposure* occurs when exposure is six to 24 hours, and can be either a land based or water immersion experience.

3. *Chronic exposure* involves long-term cooling. It generally occurs on land and lasts more than 24 hours.

Types of Hypothermia

A victim's core body temperature determines the type of hypothermia. To take the temperature, you need a low-reading thermometer, not the standard rectal thermometer, which is calibrated from 94 to 108°F. The recommended type is a rectal thermometer capable of

---

TABLE 9-1 Wind-Chill Factor

Estimated Wind Speed (in MPH)	Actual Thermometer Reading (°F.)											
	50	40	30	20	10	0	−10	−20	−30	−40	−50	−60
	Equivalent Temperature (°F.)											
calm	50	40	30	20	10	0	−10	−20	−30	−40	−50	−60
5	48	37	27	16	6	−5	−15	−26	−36	−47	−57	−68
10	40	28	16	4	−9	−24	−33	−46	−58	−70	−83	−95
15	36	22	9	−5	−18	−32	−45	−58	−72	−85	−99	−112
20	32	18	4	−10	−25	−39	−53	−67	−82	−96	−110	−124
25	30	16	0	−15	−29	−44	−59	−74	−88	−104	−118	−133
30	25	13	−2	−18	−33	−48	−63	−79	−94	−109	−125	−140
35	27	11	−4	−20	−35	−51	−67	−82	−98	−113	−129	−145
40	26	10	−6	−21	−37	−53	−69	−85	−100	−116	−132	−148

(Wind speeds greater than 40 mph have little additional effect.)

Little danger (for properly clothed person). Maximum danger of false sense of security.

Increasing danger. (Flesh may freeze within 1 minute.)

Great danger. (Flesh may freeze within 30 seconds.)

Your Winter Wardrobe

	Advantages	Disadvantages	Wear In
WOOL	Stretches without damage; insulates well even when wet	Heavy weight; absorbs moisture; may irritate skin	Layer 1, 2 or 3
COTTON	Comfortable and lightweight	Absorbs moisture	Layer 1 (for inactive people) or 2
SILK	Extremely lightweight and durable; very good insulator; washes well.	More expensive; does not transfer moisture quickly	Layer 1
POLY-PROPYLENE	Lightweight; transfers moisture quickly and dries quickly	Does not insulate well; low melting point; surface may pill up	Layer 1 or 2 (for active people)
DOWN	Durable, lightweight; most effective insulator by weight	Expensive; loses insulative quality when wet; difficult to dry	Layer 2 or 3 (especially in dry, extreme cold)
NYLON	Lightweight; wind- and water-resistant; durable	May not allow perspiration to evaporate; low melting point; flammable	Layer 3
SYNTHETIC POLYESTER INSULATION	Does not absorb moisture, therefore insulates even when wet	Heavier than down; does not compress as well	Layer 2 or 3 (especially in wet weather)

Source: National Safety Council Family Safety & Health

■ HYPOTHERMIA ■

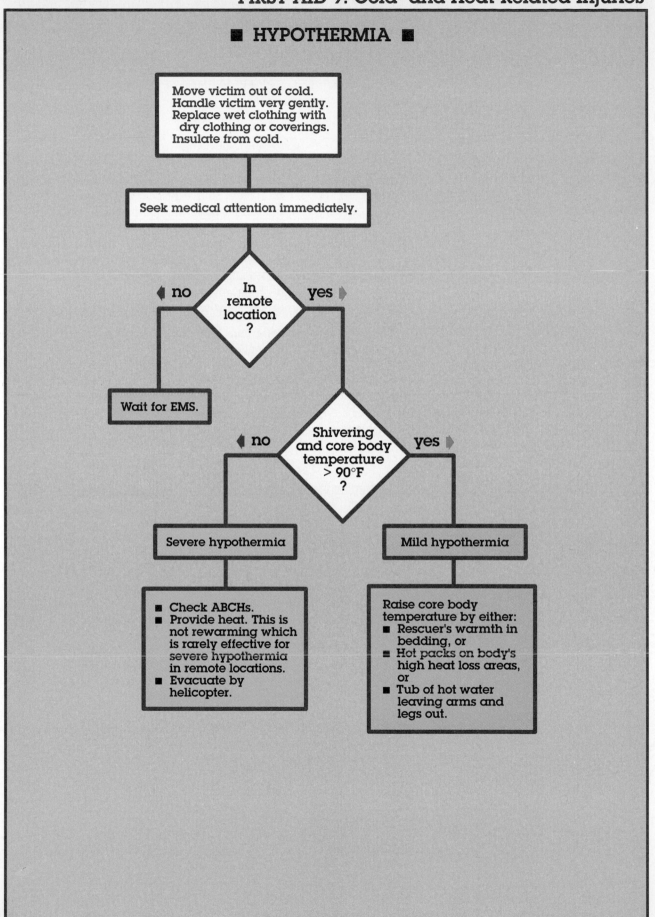

Move victim out of cold.
Handle victim very gently.
Replace wet clothing with
dry clothing or coverings.
Insulate from cold.

Seek medical attention immediately.

In remote location ?

◀ no   yes ▶

Wait for EMS.

Shivering and core body temperature > 90°F ?

◀ no   yes ▶

Severe hypothermia

Mild hypothermia

- Check ABCHs.
- Provide heat. This is not rewarming which is rarely effective for severe hypothermia in remote locations.
- Evacuate by helicopter.

Raise core body temperature by either:
- Rescuer's warmth in bedding, or
- Hot packs on body's high heat loss areas, or
- Tub of hot water leaving arms and legs out.

Lowest Body Temperature

There are three recorded cases of people who survived body temperatures as low as 60.8°F. Dorothy Mae Stevens was found in an alley in Chicago on February 1, 1951. Vickie Mary David of Milwaukee, Wisconsin, at age 2 years 1 month was admitted to the Evangelical Hospital, Marshalltown, Iowa, January 21, 1956, after having been found unconscious on the floor of an unheated house. Michael Trode, aged 2, was found in the snow near his home in Milwaukee, Wisconsin, on January 19, 1985. All three had a temperature of 60.8°F when found. People may die of hypothermia with body temperatures of 95 degrees F.

—*Guinness Book of World Records*

reading temperatures between 84 to 108°F. These thermometers are hard to find.

1. *Mild* (above 90°F). Shivering, slurred speech, memory lapses, and fumbling hands. Victims frequently stumble and stagger. They are usually conscious and can talk. While many people suffer cold hands and feet, victims of mild hypothermia experience cold abdomens and backs.

2. *Profound* (below 90°F). Shivering has stopped. Muscles may become stiff and rigid, similar to rigor mortis. The victim's skin has a blue appearance and doesn't respond to pain; pulse and respirations slow down, and pupils dilate. The victim appears to be dead. Fifty to 80% of all profound hypothermic victims die.

First Aid

1. General Suggestions
   Stop further heat loss by doing the following:
   a. Get the victim out of the cold environment.
   b. Have a source of heat (e.g., stove, fire).
   c. Add insulation beneath and around the victim. Cover the victim's head since 50% of the body's heat loss is through the head.
   d. Replace wet clothing with dry clothing.
   e. Handle the victim gently.
   f. Treat any injuries.

2. Mild Hypothermia (core temperature above 90°F)
   Raise core temperature by one of the following means available:
   a. Use a tub of hot water (no greater than 106°F) or electric blanket. *Leave victim's arms and legs out.*
   b. Place hot packs against the body's areas of high heat loss (e.g., head, neck, chest, and groin). Do not burn the victim.

TABLE 9-2 Heat Index

Relative Humidity	Air Temperature										
	70	75	80	85	90	95	100	105	110	115	120
	Apparent Temperature*										
0%	64	69	73	78	83	87	91	95	99	103	107
10%	65	70	75	80	85	90	95	100	105	111	116
20%	66	72	77	82	87	93	99	105	112	120	130
30%	67	73	78	84	90	96	104	113	123	135	148
40%	68	74	79	86	93	101	110	123	137	151	
50%	69	75	81	88	96	107	120	135	150		
60%	70	76	82	90	100	114	132	149			
70%	70	77	85	93	106	124	144				
80%	71	78	86	97	113	136					
90%	71	79	88	102	122						
100%	72	80	91	108							

*Degrees Fahrenheit.

Above 130°F = heat stroke imminent
105°–130°F = heat exhaustion and heat cramps likely and heat stroke with long exposure and activity
90°–105°F = heat exhaustion and heat cramps with long exposure and activity
80°–90°F = fatigue during exposure and activity

Source: National Weather Service

c. Have a rescuer lie trunk to trunk with the victim in a sleeping bag.

3. Profound Hypothermia (core temperature below 90°F)

a. Do *not* rewarm the victim if he or she can be transported within 12 hours. Keep the victim from getting colder.

b. Do *not* jostle or jolt the victim during transportation.

c. *Avoid* CPR unless the victim has no pulse. Start CPR immediately in near-drowning cases. Pulses are difficult to detect so take a full minute to check them. CPR could actually induce cardiac arrest. Once CPR is begun, it should be continued until arrival at a medical facility. Hypothermic victims have survived after long-term CPR (unlike those with cardiac arrest from other causes).

Warm drinks have no warming effect and contain little energy. Warm drinks send a message to the brain to send more blood to the skin. Dilation of the skin's blood vessels produces a warm feeling and some heat loss since the capillaries are dilated.

Avoid cardiac arrest by observing the following guidelines:

- *Never* allow the victim to physically exert himself (i.e., no walking, climbing, etc.).
- Make *no* attempt to rapidly rewarm a profound hypothermic victim outside of a medical facility. Most circumstances require no rewarming attempts at all.
- Handle a profound hypothermic victim as carefully and gently as though every arm and leg were broken.

Cautions

- Do *not* put an unconscious victim in a bathtub.
- Do *not* give the unconscious victim anything to drink.
- Do *not* give the victim alcohol.
- Do *not* attempt to rewarm the body by rubbing the arms and legs.
- Do *not* allow the victim to move about, walk, or struggle.
- Do *not* wrap a victim in a blanket without another source of heat unless it is to protect the victim against further heat loss since such victims cannot generate sufficient heat to rewarm themselves, and blankets insulate them from the warm environment.
- Do *not* stop resuscitative attempts until the victim has been rewarmed and preferably evaluated at a medical facility.
- Do *not* rewarm the victim outside of a medical facility if he or she can be transported within

12 hours. Victims can be hypothermic for long periods of time and still recover.

- Do *not* give CPR unless the victim is pulseless. Use CPR in cases of near-drowning. Monitor pulse for a full minute.
- Do *not* rewarm extremities and body core (chest, abdomen) at the same time.

Heat-Related Emergencies

There are two types of major heat illness—heat stroke and heat exhaustion, and two types of minor heat illness—heat cramps and heat syncope.

Heat Stroke (sunstroke)

Heat stroke is the most dangerous heat-related emergency. The death rate from this condition approaches 50%, even with appropriate medical care. Untreated victims always die. Heat stroke happens when the body is subjected to more heat than it can handle.

Types of Heat Stroke

- *Classic.* This type affects the elderly, chronically ill, obese, alcoholic, diabetic, and those with circulatory problems. It results from a combination of a hot environment and body mechanisms incapable of handling heat exposure.

Highest Body Temperature

Sustained body temperatures of much over 109°F are normally incompatible with life, although recoveries after readings of 111°F have been noted. Marathon runners in hot weather attain 105.8°F.

Willie Jones, 52 years old, was admitted to Grady Memorial Hospital, Atlanta, Georgia, on July 10, 1980, with heat stroke on a day when the temperature reached 90°F with 44% humidity. His temperature was found to be 115.7°F.

—*Guinness Book of World Records*

Highest Temperature Endured

The highest dry-air temperature endured by naked men in U.S. Air Force experiments in 1960 was 400°F and for heavily clothed men 500°F. (Steaks require only 325°F.) Temperatures of 284°F have been found quite bearable in sauna baths.

—*Guinness Book of World Records*

- *Exertional.* This type affects a healthy individual when strenuously working or playing in a warm environment.

Signs and Symptoms:

- Unconscious
- Hot skin. Victims do not sweat because the sweating mechanism is overwhelmed. Half the victims with exertional heat stroke may have sweat on the skin since they are progressing from heat exhaustion (having sweaty skin) into heat stroke.
- High body temperature
- Rapid pulse and breathing
- Weakness, dizziness, headache

First Aid

Heat stroke is a true emergency! If normal temperature is not promptly restored, permanent disability or even death will occur.

- Move the victim to a cool place. Remove heavy clothing; light clothing can be left in place.
- Immediately cool the victim by any available means. Because ice is rarely available, an effective method is to wrap the victim in wet towels or sheets, and fan the victim. Keep the cloths wet with cool water. If using ice, place ice packs at areas with abundant blood supply (e.g., neck, armpits, and groin). Continue cooling the victim until his or her temperature drops to 102°F. Stop at this point to prevent seizures and hypothermia. Keep head and shoulders slightly elevated.
- Monitor the ABCs and treat accordingly.
- Care for seizures, if they occur.
- All heat stroke victims need hospitalization so seek medical attention as fast as possible. Continue cooling en route.

Heat Exhaustion

Heat exhaustion results from either excessive perspiration or the inadequate replacement of water lost by sweating. It is less critical than heat stroke, but it requires prompt attention because it can progress to heat stroke if left untreated.

Signs and Symptoms

- Heavy sweating
- Weakness
- Fast pulse
- Normal body temperature
- Headache and dizziness
- Nausea and vomiting

TABLE 9–3 Heat-related Emergencies

Indicators	Heat Cramps (least serious)	Heat Exhaustion (serious)	Heat Stroke (most serious)
Muscle cramps	Yes	No	No
Skin	Normal, moist-warm	Cold, clammy	Hot, dry
Temperature	Normal	Normal or slightly elevated	>105° F.
Loss of consciousness	Seldom	Sometimes	Usually
Perspiration	Heavy	Heavy	Little or none
First aid	Move to cool place.	Move to cool place.	Move to cool place.
	Rest affected muscle.	Elevate legs.	Elevate head and shoulders.
	Give a lot of cold water.	Cool victim.	Immediately cool victim.
	Do *not* massage.	If no improvement in 30 minutes, seek medical attention.	Immediately transport to medical facility.
			Monitor ABCs.
			Heat stroke is life-threatening!

First Aid

- Move the victim to a cool place.
- Keep victim lying down with legs up.
- Cool the victim by applying cold packs or wet towels or cloths. Fan the victim.
- Give the victim cold water if he or she is fully conscious.
- If no improvement is noted within 30 minutes, seek medical attention.

Heat Cramps

Heat cramps are painful muscle spasms in the arms or legs. They may occur when an excessive amount of body fluid is lost through sweating. Controversy exists regarding what type of liquid to drink—plain water, a commercial sports drink, or a saltwater solution. The body loses more water than electrolytes (sodium, potassium, etc.) during exercise. Experts generally agree that the primary need for those sweating in hot environments is to replace the water lost from heavy sweating, rather than the electrolytes. However, mildly salted water (¼ to 1 level teaspoon in 1 quart of water) or electrolyte drink can be given.

Routine use of salt tablets to prevent heat cramps is no longer recommended since they can induce high blood pressure and hinder adjustment to heat.

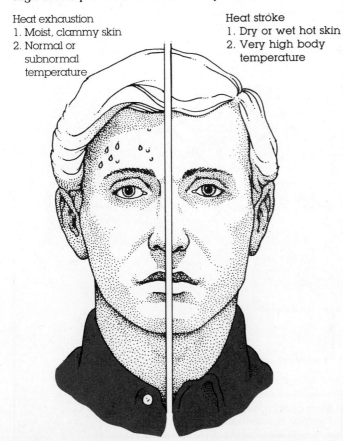

Heat exhaustion
1. Moist, clammy skin
2. Normal or subnormal temperature

Heat stroke
1. Dry or wet hot skin
2. Very high body temperature

Signs and symptoms of heat stroke and heat exhaustion

Signs and Symptoms

- Severe cramping, usually affecting arms or legs
- Abdominal cramping

First Aid

- Move the victim to a cool place.
- Stretch the cramping muscle.
- Give victim a lot of cold water or sports drink.
- Do *not* massage since it rarely provides relief and may even worsen the pain.

Heat Syncope

This condition resembles fainting and is usually self-correcting. Victims who are not nauseated can drink water. First aid consists of having the victim lie down in a cool place.

■ HEAT-RELATED EMERGENCIES ■

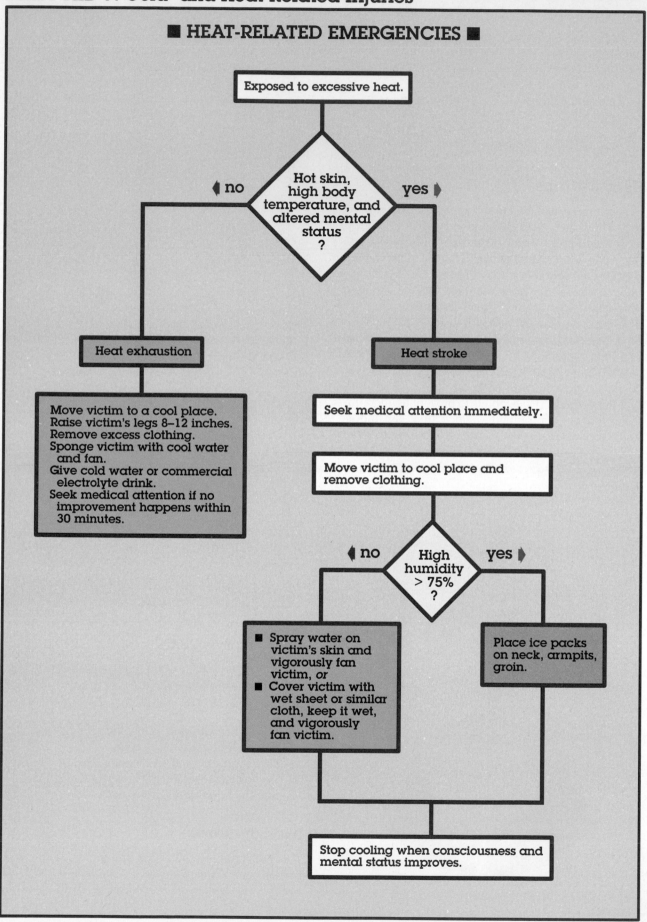

Exposed to excessive heat.

Hot skin, high body temperature, and altered mental status ?

◄ no   yes ►

Heat exhaustion

Heat stroke

Move victim to a cool place.
Raise victim's legs 8–12 inches.
Remove excess clothing.
Sponge victim with cool water and fan.
Give cold water or commercial electrolyte drink.
Seek medical attention if no improvement happens within 30 minutes.

Seek medical attention immediately.

Move victim to cool place and remove clothing.

High humidity > 75% ?

◄ no   yes ►

■ Spray water on victim's skin and vigorously fan victim, or
■ Cover victim with wet sheet or similar cloth, keep it wet, and vigorously fan victim.

Place ice packs on neck, armpits, groin.

Stop cooling when consciousness and mental status improves.

■ ACTIVITY 1 ■
Frostbite

Mark each action yes (Y) or no (N)

Which of the following actions are proper first aid for frostbite?

1. ____ Rewarm a frostbitten part by exposing it to a fire or open flame.

2. ____ Rewarm a frostbitten part by using warm water (102–106°F).

3. ____ Placing frostbitten hands in another person's armpits is as effective as using warm water.

4. ____ Rub the frostbitten part to restore circulation.

5. ____ Rub the frostbitten area with snow.

6. ____ A victim with frozen lower extremities should be carried, if possible, to the nearest medical facility.

7. ____ If a victim with a severely frostbitten foot cannot be carried to medical aid, keep the part frozen and assist him in walking.

8. ____ Break any blisters that have formed.

■ ACTIVITY 2 ■
Hypothermia

Check (✓) the appropriate action(s).

Which of the following actions are proper first aid for hypothermia?

1. ____ Give hot coffee or chocolate to rewarm a victim.

2. ____ Treat the victim gently.

For mild hypothermia:

5. ____ Rewarm the arms and legs first since they were affected first and are accessible.

6. ____ Add heat to the head, neck, chest, and groin first.

For profound hypothermia:

9. ____ Check breathing and pulse for at least one full minute.

3. ____ Replace wet clothing with dry clothing.

4. ____ Get the victim out of the cold environment.

7. ____ Use a tub of hot water, but leave the victim's arms and legs out.

8. ____ Use rescuer's body heat against the victim's body while both are in a sleeping bag.

10. ____ Quickly rewarm the victim even if outside of a medical facility.

■ ACTIVITY 3 ■
Heat-Related Injuries

Choose the best answer.

On a hot day a man complains of pain in his legs and arms. Which of the following should you do?

1. ____ **A.** Give him a lot of cold water.
   B. Make a saltwater drink by adding 1 teaspoon of salt to 1 glass of water.

2. ____ **A.** Massage the cramping muscle.
   C. Rest the cramping muscle.

Mark each sign HE (heat exhaustion) or HS (heat stroke)

1. ____ skin: hot, dry or wet

2. ____ skin: cool, clammy

3. ____ sweating excessively

4. ____ sweating absent

5. ____ unconscious

Choose the best techniques.

A woman has hot, dry, red skin. Which *two* of the following cooling techniques could you use to quickly reduce her body temperature?

1. ____ Apply cold towels to her back.

2. ____ Place her feet and hands in buckets of cold water.

3. ____ Wrap the victim in wet towels or sheets and fan her.

4. ____ Apply cold, wet towels to the neck, armpits, head, and groin.

5. ____ Apply cold, wet towels around her wrists and ankles.

10

Bone, Joint, and Muscle Injuries*

■ Fractures ■ Dislocations ■ Spinal Injuries ■
■ Ankle Injuries ■ Muscle Injuries ■

Fractures

The terms **fracture** and **broken bone** have the same meaning—break or crack in a bone. Fractures are classified as being **open** (when the skin is broken and bleeds externally) or **closed** (when the skin has not been broken).

Fracture Classification

- **Open (compound) fracture.** The overlaying skin has been damaged or broken. The wound can be produced either by the bone protruding through the skin or by a direct blow cutting the skin at the time of the fracture. The bone may not always be seen in the wound. Any broken bone which is covered by damaged skin is classified as an open fracture.
- **Closed (simple) fracture.** The skin has not been broken and no wound exists anywhere near the fracture site. Open fractures are more serious than closed fractures because of greater blood loss and greater chance of infection.

Signs and Symptoms

- **Swelling.** Caused by bleeding; it occurs rapidly after a fracture.
- **Deformity.** This is not always obvious. Compare the injured with the uninjured opposite part when checking for deformity.

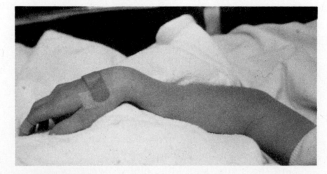

Forearm fracture

Source: Based upon American Academy of Orthopaedic Surgeons protocols.

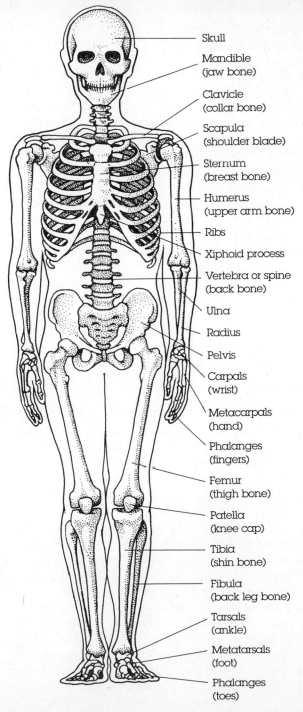

Skull

Mandible
(jaw bone)

Clavicle
(collar bone)

Scapula
(shoulder blade)

Sternum
(breast bone)

Humerus
(upper arm bone)

Ribs

Xiphoid process

Vertebra or spine
(back bone)

Ulna

Radius

Pelvis

Carpals
(wrist)

Metacarpals
(hand)

Phalanges
(fingers)

Femur
(thigh bone)

Patella
(knee cap)

Tibia
(shin bone)

Fibula
(back leg bone)

Tarsals
(ankle)

Metatarsals
(foot)

Phalanges
(toes)

Bones of the body

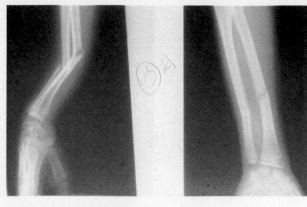

X-rays of victim with forearm fracture. One shows before setting; the other is after.

- **Pain and tenderness.** Commonly found only at the injury site. The victim will usually be able to point to the site of the pain. A useful procedure for detecting fractures is to gently feel along the bones; complaints about pain or tenderness serve as a reliable sign of a fracture.
- **Loss of use.** Inability to use the injured part. "Guarding" occurs because when motion produces pain, the victim will refuse to use it. However, sometimes the victim is able to move the limb with little or no pain.
- **Grating sensation.** Do *not* move the injured limb as an attempt to see if a grating sensation (called **crepitus**) can be felt and even sometimes heard when the broken bone ends rub together.
- **History of the injury.** Suspect a fracture whenever severe accidents (e.g., motor-vehicle accidents, falls) happen. The victim may have heard or felt the bone snap.

First Aid

The first aid procedures listed here are basic guidelines.

- Treat any life-threatening emergencies. Broken bones (except spinal or pelvic breaks) seldom present an immediate threat to life.
- Treat the victim for shock.
- Determine what happened and the location of pain, numbness, tingling.
- Gently remove clothing surrounding the injured area. Do *not* move the injured area unless necessary. Cut clothing at the seams if necessary. Check for swelling, deformity, tenderness, guarding, and open wounds.
- Control bleeding and cover all wounds before splinting. In open fractures, do *not* attempt to push bone ends back beneath the skin surface. Simply cover them with a sterile dressing.
- Check for a pulse, sensations, and capillary refill. Compare area with an uninjured part.

    A quick nerve and circulatory exam is very important. Fractures can injure nerves.

Check for nerve damage by checking for sensations and asking the victim to flex the hand or foot, depending upon the fracture location.

A quick circulatory exam is important because prolonged loss of blood to an extremity rapidly results in irreversible damage. Check the radial pulse at the wrist and the dorsalis pedis pulse in the foot. About one person in five has no detectable dorsalis pedis pulse, so if it is absent, check for a posterior tibial pulse. (The dorsalis pedis pulse is located on top of the foot, whereas the posterior tibial pulse can be found behind the inside ankle bone.) If you can not detect a pulse, obtain medical assistance immediately. Capillary refilling can also be used as a check for circulation. Do *not* wait to see whether circulation will return before getting help.

If the victim's hand or foot is cold, pale, and pulseless, and medical care is more than 15 minutes away, many experts recommend realigning the limb with gentle manual traction. This involves pulling *gently* in line with the normal bone position. If there is great pain or resistance to this gentle traction, splint the fracture as it is.

- All fractures should be splinted before the victim is moved unless the victim's life is endangered. When splinting possible fractures, immobilize the joints above and below the fracture site. Splinting helps prevent further injury to soft tissues, blood vessels, or nerves from sharp bone fragments and relieves pain by stopping motion at the fracture site. Keep the fingers and toes exposed in order to check circulation even though they may be included within a splint.
- Several commonly available materials can form splints. An arm sling and swathe, a pillow, cardboard, boards, newspapers, blankets—even tying the injured part to an uninjured part—all serve well as splints. Padded splints prevent pressure to nerves and skin.
- Severely deformed fractures should be realigned before splinting if a pulse is absent. This helps preserve or restore circulation. This involves gently pulling in line with the normal bone position. Explain to the victim that straightening the fracture may cause momentary pain, but that it will stop once the fracture is straightened and splinted. If the victim shows increased pain or resistance, splint the extremity in the deformed position. Do *not* straighten dislocations or any fractures involving the spine, shoulder, elbow, wrist, or knee.
- Never reduce or replace open fractures. Cover the wound with a sterile dressing. Then apply the appropriate splint.

- If the victim has a possible spinal injury as well as an extremity injury, the spinal injury takes precedence. Splinting the spine is always a problem. Immobilize the spine with rolled blankets or similar objects placed on either side of the neck and torso. In most cases it is best to wait until an ambulance arrives with trained personnel and proper equipment to handle spinal injuries.
- Position the injured part slightly above the heart's level to help control swelling and pain. Cold packs help control swelling and pain but avoid overuse because of frostbite.
- Most fractures do not require rapid transportation. An exception involves the arm or leg without a pulse, which means insufficient blood is being provided for the affected arm or leg. This necessitates seeking immediate medical attention.
- If in doubt, splint and treat as if there were a fracture.
- Analgesics can help reduce the pain associated with an injury. Do *not* give aspirin or acetaminophen if the victim cannot tolerate it. Cold packs can also help reduce pain.

Dislocations

Dislocations occur in a joint when it is pushed beyond its normal range of motion.

Signs and Symptoms

- Deformity of a joint
- Severe pain in a joint
- Swelling around the joint
- Discoloration around the joint
- Inability to move the injured area
- Appearance differing from comparable uninjured joint

First Aid

- Check the pulse, sensation, and capillary refill of the injured extremity (compare with uninjured part).
- Splint as if a fracture.
- Do *not* replace the joint since nerve and blood vessel damage could happen.

Types of Splints

Any device used to immobilize a fracture or dislocation is a splint. Splint by using:

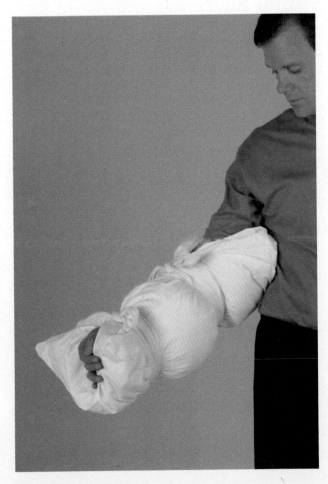

Types of splints.   Commercial (air splint)   Improvised (pillow)

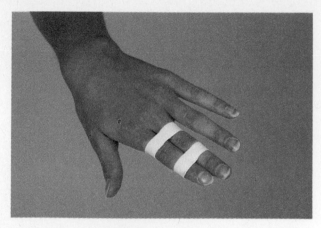

Using victim's body as a splint

- **Improvised splint.** Use pillow, folded newspaper, magazine, cardboard, wooden board, or any other object that can provide stability.
- **Victim's body.** Tie injured part to uninjured part (e.g., injured finger to adjacent finger; legs tied together; injured arm tied to chest).
- **Commercial splint.** Use wire splints, air splints, SAM Splints™

Spinal Injuries

The spine is a column of vertebrae stacked one on the next from the skull's base to the tail bone. Each vertebra has a hollow center through which the spinal cord passes. The spinal cord consists of long tracts of nerves that join the brain with all body organs and parts.

If a broken spinal column pinches spinal nerves, paralysis can result. All unconscious victims should be treated as though they had spinal injuries. All conscious victims sustaining injuries from falls, diving accidents, auto accidents, or cave-in should be carefully checked for spine injuries before moving them.

A mistake in handling a spinal injured victim could mean a lifetime in a wheelchair or bed for the victim. Suspect a spinal injury in all severe accidents.

Signs and Symptoms

- Head injuries serve as a clue since the head may have been snapped suddenly in one or more directions, endangering the spine. About 15% to 20% of head injured victims also have neck and spinal cord injuries.
- Painful movement of arms and/or legs
- Numbness, tingling, weakness, or burning sensation in arms or legs
- Loss of bowel or bladder control
- Paralysis to arms and/or legs
- Deformity; odd-looking angle of the victim's head and neck

Ask the conscious victim the following questions:

- **Is there pain?** Neck injuries (cervical) radiate pain to the arms; upper back injuries (thoracic) radiate pain around the ribs and into the chest; lower back injuries (lumbar) usually radiate pain down the legs. Often the victim describes the pain as "electric."
- **Can you move your feet?** Ask the victim to move his or her foot against your hand. If the victim cannot perform this movement or if the movement is extremely weak against your hand, the victim may have injured the spinal cord.
- **Can you move your fingers?** Moving the fingers is a sign that nerve pathways are intact. Ask the victim to grip your hand. A strong grip indicates that a spinal cord injury is unlikely.

For an unconscious victim:

- Look for cuts, bruises, and deformities.
- Test responses by pinching the victim's hands (either palm or back) and foot (sole or top of the bare foot). No reaction could mean spinal cord damage.
- Ask others about what happened. If not sure about a possible spinal injury, assume that the victim has one until proven otherwise.

First Aid

- Check and monitor the airway, breathing, and circulation, and treat accordingly. Do *not* use the head tilt because it would move the neck. Instead, jut the jaw forward by placing the fingers on the corners of the jaw and pushing forward (known as the "jaw thrust"). Keep the head and neck still.
- First aiders should normally wait for the Emergency Medical Service (EMS) to transport the victim because of their training and equipment. Victims with suspected spine injuries will require cervical collars and immobilization on a spine board. It is better to do nothing than to mishandle these victims. Splinting requires at least two trained people. Do *not* attempt to splint a victim by yourself.
- Stabilize the victim against any movement. Do *not* move the neck to reposition it except when danger is present (e.g., smoking or burning car or burning building). Bring help to the victim, *not* the victim to the help.
- The victim must be immobilized. Tell the victim not to move, if he or she is conscious. Place objects on either side of the head to prevent it from rolling from side to side.
- Victims in water with potential neck or back injury must be floated gently to shore. Before removal from the water, the victim must be secured to a backboard.

■ FRACTURES ■

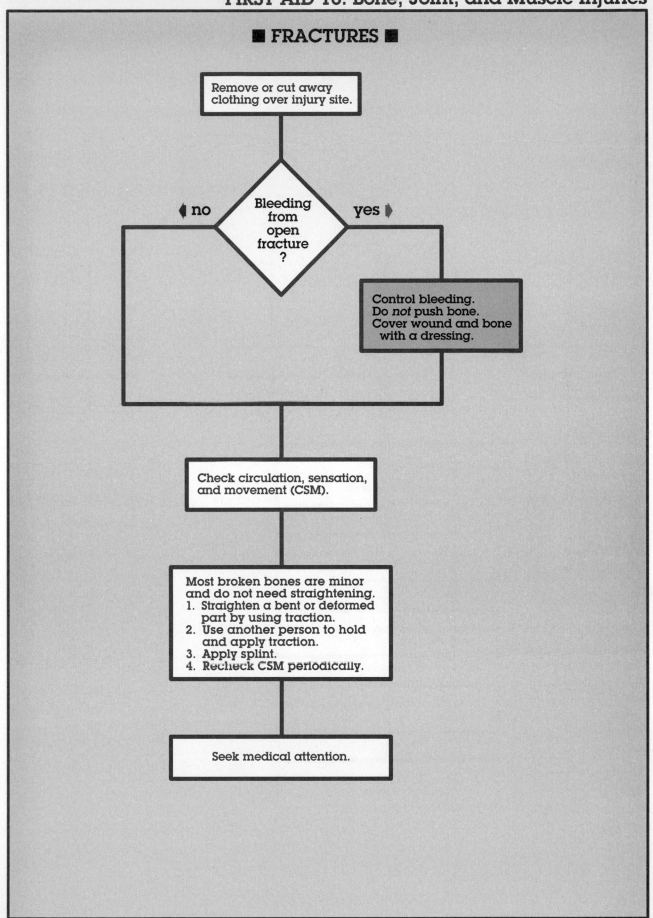

Remove or cut away clothing over injury site.

Bleeding from open fracture?

◄ no   yes ▶

Control bleeding.
Do *not* push bone.
Cover wound and bone with a dressing.

Check circulation, sensation, and movement (CSM).

Most broken bones are minor and do not need straightening.
1. Straighten a bent or deformed part by using traction.
2. Use another person to hold and apply traction.
3. Apply splint.
4. Recheck CSM periodically.

Seek medical attention.

■ SPRAINS, STRAINS, CONTUSIONS, DISLOCATIONS ■

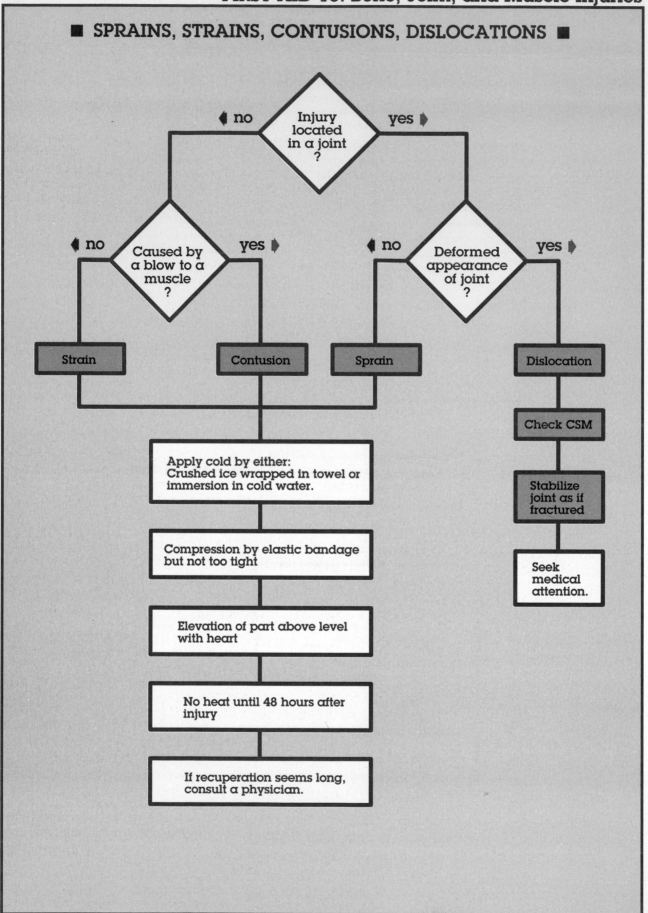

■ SPINAL INJURIES ■

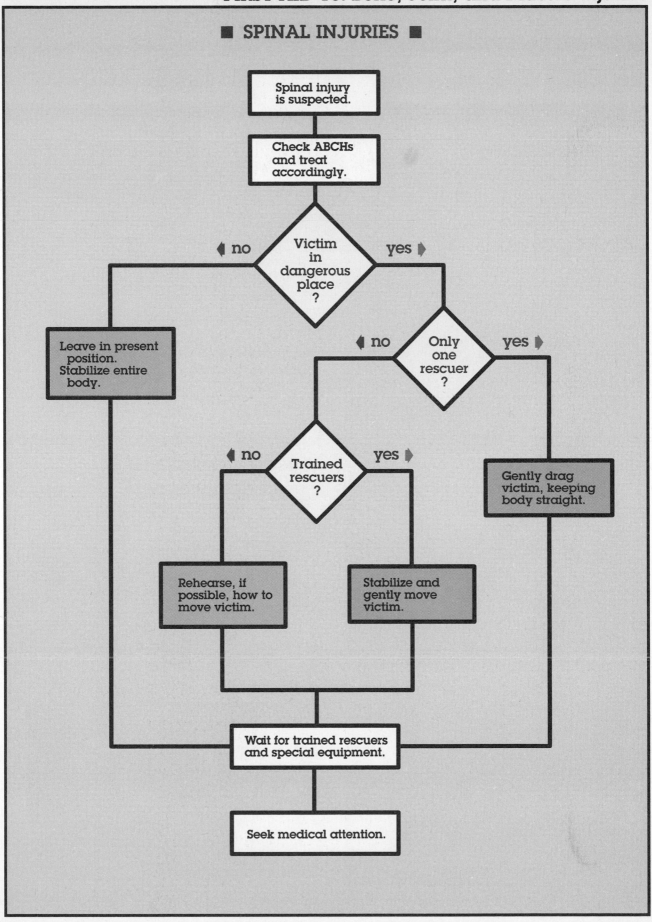

Spinal injury
is suspected.

Check ABCHs
and treat
accordingly.

Victim
in
dangerous
place
?

◀ no   yes ▶

Leave in present
position.
Stabilize entire
body.

Only
one
rescuer
?

◀ no   yes ▶

Gently drag
victim, keeping
body straight.

Trained
rescuers
?

◀ no   yes ▶

Rehearse, if
possible, how to
move victim.

Stabilize and
gently move
victim.

Wait for trained rescuers
and special equipment.

Seek medical attention.

CONSCIOUS VICTIM—UPPER EXTREMITY CHECKS

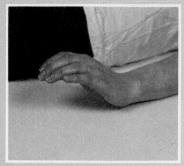

1. Victim wiggles fingers.

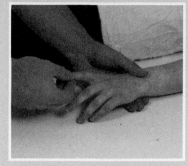

2. Rescuer touches fingers.

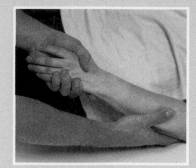

3. Victim squeezes rescuer's hand.

CONSCIOUS VICTIM—LOWER EXTREMITY CHECKS

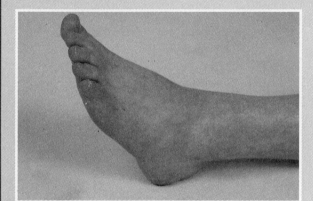

1. Victim wiggles toes.

2. Rescuer touches toes.

3. Victim pushes foot against rescuer's hand.

Victim's failure to perform may mean spinal cord injury!

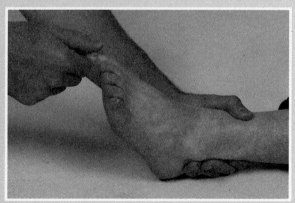

1.

UNCONSCIOUS VICTIM

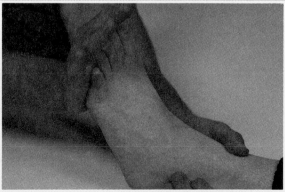
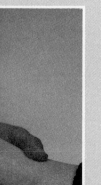

2.

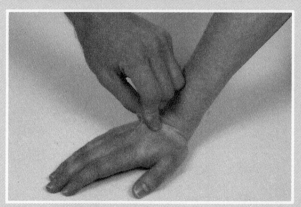

1. Pinch hand.

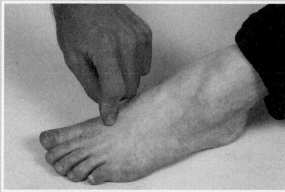

2. Pinch foot.

3.

Ankle Injuries

The ankle frequently gets injured and it should *not* be handled casually. Careless treatment can have consequences that include a lifelong disability. In some cases, the damage requires surgical correction.

Signs and Symptoms

It is difficult to tell the difference between a severely sprained and a fractured ankle. Treat the injury as a fracture until you can get the advice of a physician.

The following suggestions, though not 100% accurate, may help determine whether the injury is a sprained or fractured ankle:

1. Ask the victim, "Did you try to stand on it?" Putting some weight on the ankle may hurt a little, but if the victim is able to do that and take four or more steps, most likely the ankle is sprained. If it is broken, the victim will not even want to try putting any weight on it, and if walking is tried, no more than four steps will be taken.

2. Press your fingers along the ankle bones. Pain and tenderness over the bones at either the: (a) back edge or tip of either of the ankle knob bones (malleolus bones) or (b) midfoot's outside bone (fifth metatarsal) or on the inside bones may indicate a broken bone.

3. Ankle sprains tend to swell only on one side of the foot. This swelling is usually on the outside of the ankle since most sprains damage the outside (lateral) of the ankle. Swelling on both sides of the ankle usually accompanies a broken bone.

First Aid

Remember the mnemonic **RICE: R**est, **I**ce, **C**ompression, **E**levation as a guide to sprained ankle injuries.

- **R** stands for rest.
- **I** stands for the application of cold, which causes constriction of the blood vessels. This decreases the amount of bleeding, swelling, and pain.

  Cold is available from ice, commercially prepared ice packs, frozen food cans, drinking fountains, etc. The earlier cold is applied, the better. Try using crushed ice rather than ice cubes since crushed ice contours to the shape of the ankle better.

  Do *not* place ice directly on the skin except in periodic ice massages because it can cause frostbite. Place a towel or washcloth between the ice pack and skin.

  Applying cold for short periods of time does not cool deeper tissues—it only lowers skin temperature. The cold application should be continued for at least 20-30 minutes. This should occur about three times during the first 24 hours after the injury.

  A common mistake is the early use of heat. Heat causes swelling and pain if applied too early. A minimum of 24 hours and preferably 48–72 hours should pass before applying any heat.

- **C** represents compression. Swelling is like glue and can lock up a joint within hours. It is important to prevent swelling by using cold promptly, and also make the swelling recede as quickly as possible with a compression (elastic) bandage.

  Some experts believe elastic bandages are often applied too tightly. Do *not* apply the bandage too firmly. Toes should be checked periodically for skin discoloration and coldness, indicating that the bandage has been applied too tightly. Comparing the toes of the injured foot with those of the uninjured foot is also suggested. Pain, tingling, loss of sensation, and loss of pulses also indicate impaired circulation. Loosen the elastic bandage if any of these signs or symptoms appear.

  To counteract swelling, take any soft, pliable material (e.g., sock, T-shirt) and either fold or cut it into the shape of a horseshoe. Place this "horseshoe" around the ankle bone knob on the injured side with the curved part down. Then place a figure-of-eight wrap around the ankle covering the "horseshoe" and foot with an elastic bandage. This technique applies compression to the soft tissue areas, not just the ankle bone and tendon.

- **E** stands for elevation. To further reduce swelling and bleeding, tell the victim to elevate the ankle about six inches for the first 24 to 48 hours. Some medical experts say, "Keep the foot higher than the knee and the knee higher than the heart." Avoid any weight on the ankle. Some victims should consider crutches.

  Swelling and pain should begin to subside within 48 hours, and the ankle should be nearly normal within 10 days. If the injury is not healing, consult with a physician.

  If a fracture is suspected, immobilize the ankle with a pillow splint and seek medical attention. Controversy exists regarding whether or not to take off a shoe. Those favoring leaving the shoe on believe it acts as a splint and helps in retarding swelling. Others believe taking off the shoe allows a better examination, including checking the foot's pulse and temperature. Moreover, if a shoe or boot is left on, the swelling may reduce circulation in the foot.

■ ANKLE INJURIES ■

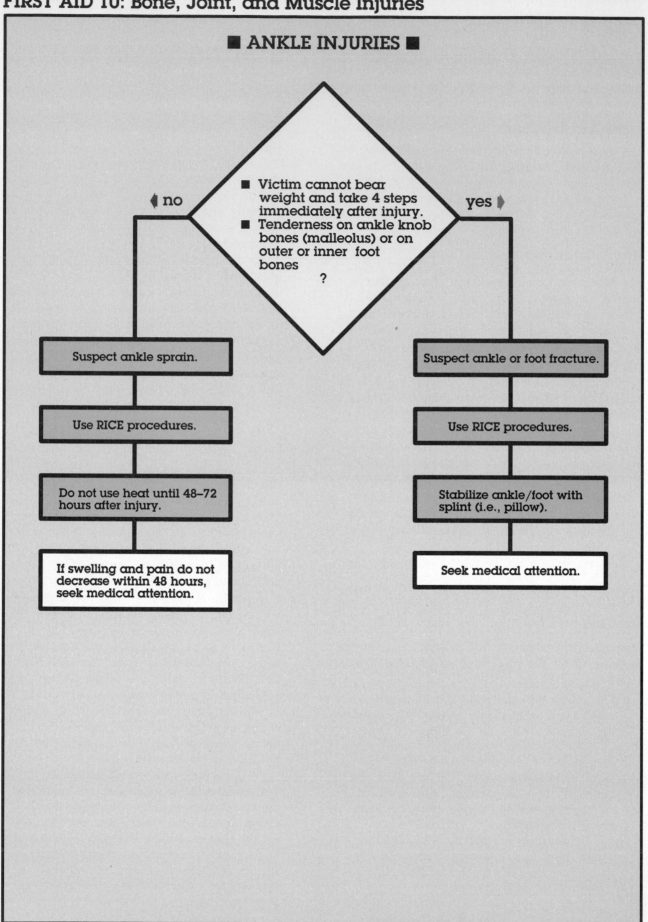

Victim cannot bear weight and take 4 steps immediately after injury.

Tenderness on ankle knob bones (malleolus) or on outer or inner foot bones ?

no →

Suspect ankle sprain.

Use RICE procedures.

Do not use heat until 48–72 hours after injury.

If swelling and pain do not decrease within 48 hours, seek medical attention.

yes →

Suspect ankle or foot fracture.

Use RICE procedures.

Stabilize ankle/foot with splint (i.e., pillow).

Seek medical attention.

Muscle Injuries

Though muscle injuries pose no real emergency, first aiders have ample opportunities to care for them.

Muscle Strains

A muscle strain, also known as muscle pull, occurs when the muscle is stretched beyond its normal range of motion, resulting in a muscle fiber tear.

Signs and Symptoms

- A sharp pain immediately after the injury
- Extreme tenderness when area is felt
- Disfigurement (indentation, cavity, or bump)
- Severe weakness and loss of function of the injured part
- The sound of a snap when the tissue is torn

Muscle Contusions

Muscle contusions result from a blow to a muscle. This injury is also known as a bruise.

First Aid for Muscle Strains and Contusions

Even though the rest, ice, compression, and elevation (RICE) procedure is universally used as the first aid for muscle strains and contusions, many first aiders and even hospital emergency department personnel mistakenly treat new muscle injuries with heat packs.

- **Rest.** Do *not* use the injured part.
- **Ice.** Methods of applying cold include using crushed ice as an ice pack or immersion in cold water. The application should continue for 20 to 30 minutes, three to four times during the first day, and if possible, the second day.

    Place towels or elastic bandage between the ice or cold packs and the body to insulate against the full effects of the cold. Frostbite will not occur if ice packs are applied for limited time periods. Constant use of an ice pack is not necessary because of the lasting effect of cold to body tissue.

    The use of cold to an injured area reduces the pain, bleeding, and swelling that follow a muscle strain or contusion.
- **Compression.** A compression (elastic) bandage applied to the injured area serves to limit internal bleeding. Often, the elastic bandage is

Cryotherapy

Ice is one of the most verstile panaceas available for injuries. The use of ice or other equally cold applications to treat muscle strains, bruises, joint sprains, insect stings, and minor burns is called **cryotherapy**.

Cryotherapy is effective because cold applications reduce tissue temperature. This constricts blood vessels, helps control bleeding, and reduces pain.

Forms of Ice Therapy

- **Ice massage.** Rubbing ice cubes in a circular motion on the affected area for 7 to 10 minutes on regions with little fat (e.g., elbow, knee, ankle) and about 20 minutes in areas with more fat (e.g., leg muscles) is recommended.
- **Ice bags.** Apply a bag full of crushed ice or covered ice cube to the affected area for 10 to 30 minutes. This method penetrates and lasts longer than the ice massage.
- **Cold water immersion.** An ice slush (ice cubes or crushed ice added to a bucket of water) is useful for injuries to the hand, foot, or elbow. Allow the injured part to soak in the ice slush for 10 to 20 minutes.

- **Cold packs.** Sealed plastic pouches containing a refreezable gel are available commercially. These can get very cold, so it is important that the cold packs be wrapped in a towel and that they never be applied directly to the skin.
- **Chemical "snap packs."** These sealed pouches resemble cold packs but contain two chemical envelopes that, when squeezed, mix the chemicals. A chemical reaction produces a cooling effect. Though they don't cool as well as other methods, snap packs are convenient.

    Precautions include *not* exposing the skin to cold too long which can result in frostbite. Those with any form of cold allergy, Raynaud's phenomenon, or abnormal sensitivity to cold should avoid cryotherapy.

    Other tips when using ice or other forms of cryotherapy include the following:
- Apply ice or cold immediately after an injury.
- Raise the injured area above heart level.
- Apply ice or cold for no more than 30 minutes at a time. Repeat two to four times a day until fully recovered.

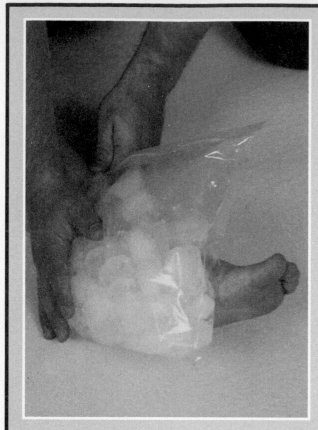

I = Ice or cold

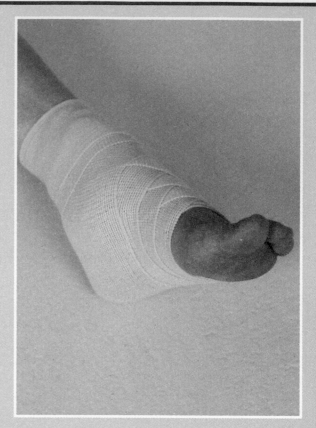

C = Compression

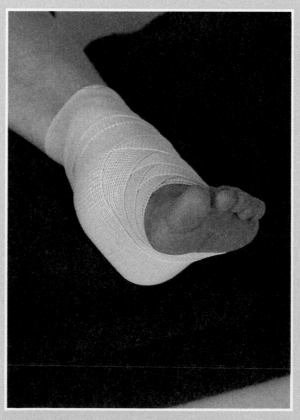

E = Elevation

applied directly to the site, the ice pack is placed over the first layer of elastic bandage wrap, and more compression elastic wrap is put over the ice. The cold with the compression limits internal bleeding common in muscle injuries. The victim should wear the elastic bandage continuously for 18 to 24 hours.

Elastic bandages may be applied too tightly, thus inhibiting blood circulation. Leave fingers and toes exposed for observing any color and temperature change. Pain, numbness, and tingling also indicate that an elastic bandage is too tight.

- *Elevation.* Elevating the injured area limits circulation to that area and helps control internal bleeding. The aim of this procedure is to get the injured part up above or even with the heart's level.

Muscle Cramps

Muscles can go into an uncontrolled spasm and contraction, resulting in severe pain and a restriction or loss of movement. Some experts believe that diet or fluid loss explains muscle cramping. Nevertheless, many different things can cause muscle cramps; no one knows all the causes.

First Aid

- Attempt to relieve a cramp by gently stretching the affected muscle. Since a muscle cramp is really an uncontrolled spasm or contraction of a muscle, a gradual lengthening of the muscle may help to lengthen those muscle fibers and relieve the cramp.
- Apply ice to the cramped muscle because it causes the muscles to relax. The exception might be during cold weather.
- Relax the affected muscle by applying pressure to it (do *not* massage).
- Pinching the upper lip hard (an accupressure technique) has been advocated for reducing calf muscle leg cramping.
- Drinking water is important because fluid deficiency appears to be a main cause. Mildly salted water (¼ to 1 level teaspoon in 1 quart of water) can also be given. Sport drinks (electrolyte drinks) can work if they do not contain a lot of sugar. Too much sugar slows fluid absorption.
- Do *not* give salt tablets. They can draw fluid out of the circulatory system and into the stomach. They can also irritate the stomach lining.

■ MUSCLE INJURIES ■

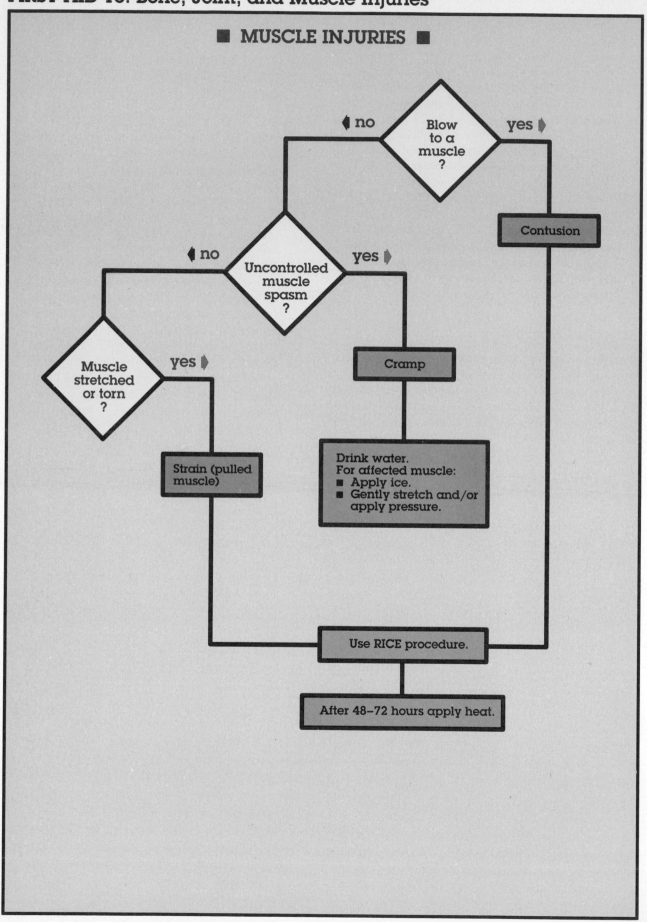

Blow to a muscle ?

◀ no   yes ▶

Contusion

Uncontrolled muscle spasm ?

◀ no   yes ▶

Cramp

Muscle stretched or torn ?

yes ▶

Strain (pulled muscle)

Drink water.
For affected muscle:
■ Apply ice.
■ Gently stretch and/or apply pressure.

Use RICE procedure.

After 48–72 hours apply heat.

■ ACTIVITY 1 ■
Fractures

Mark each procedure yes (Y) or no (N).

Which of the following are proper first aid procedures for fractures?

1. ____ Immobilize all fractures and suspected fractures before moving the victim.

2. ____ Check pulses periodically to be certain the circulation is adequate.

3. ____ Splint the joints above and below the fracture.

4. ____ In open fractures, attempt to push the bone ends back beneath the skin surface.

5. ____ Straighten fractured joints (wrist, elbow, knee, etc.)

Choose the best answer.

1. ____ A fractured elbow should be immobilized in the position in which it is found because movement may cause
   A. Further bone breakage
   B. Lower arm (radius/ulna) fracture
   C. Damage to nerves and blood vessels
   D. A dislocation

2. ____ When immobilizing a victim with a suspected fracture of the forearm, which of the following should also be immobilized by the first aider?
   A. Wrist
   B. Elbow
   C. All of the above

3. ____ When treating a victim with a suspected fracture of the lower leg, which of the following should also be immobilized?
   A. Ankle and foot
   B. Knee
   C. All of the above

4. ____ A fracture where the bone ends have pushed through the skin and have been pulled back into the skin:
   A. Is a closed fracture
   B. Is an open fracture
   C. Should not be covered with a sterile dressing to allow the first aider to view the injury
   D. Should be covered with a sterile dressing but not splinted.

5. ____ An open fracture should be treated by:
   A. Covering the fracture with a sterile dressing and applying a splint
   B. Transporting the victim without splinting
   C. Applying only a splint

6. ____ Fractures involving a joint should be immobilized:
   A. In the position it is found
   B. In the position of function
   C. With an air splint
   D. After it has been gently straightened

■ ACTIVITY 2 ■
Spinal Injuries

Check (✓) the signs and symptoms that indicate a possible spinal injury.

1. ____ Description of pain down the arms or legs
2. ____ Ability to strongly grip your hand and move a foot against your hand pressure
3. ____ A severe head injury
4. ____ Inability to move fingers and toes when asked to do so

Mark each statement true (T) or false (F).

1. ____ Do not move a victim unless extreme hazards exist (e.g., burning building or car).
2. ____ Careless moving of a victim may permanently confine him to a wheelchair.
3. ____ Move a spinal cord injured victim as quickly as possible to a medical facility.
4. ____ The head tilt can be used for non-breathing victims with spinal cord injuries.

■ ACTIVITY 3 ■
Ankle Injuries

Mark each statement true (T) or false (F).

1. ____ Telling the difference between a broken ankle and a sprained ankle can be difficult.
2. ____ The letters *RICE* represent the treatment for an ankle injury.
3. ____ When using ice, place it directly on the skin.
4. ____ A common mistake involves applying heat too soon.

5. ____ An elastic bandage, if used correctly, can help control swelling.
6. ____ Using an elastic bandage alone provides adequate compression.
7. ____ Controversy exists about whether or not to take a shoe off an injured ankle.

■ ACTIVITY 4 ■
Muscle Injuries

Mark the following statements true (T) or false (F).

1. ____ A muscle injury is a real emergency.
2. ____ Muscle strains and muscle pulls describe the same injury.
3. ____ A muscle strain can involve the tearing of a muscle.
4. ____ A blow to the muscle is also known as a bruise.
5. ____ Heat packs can initially be placed on a muscle injury to reduce pain.
6. ____ An application of cold should be left on the muscle injury for at least 20 to 30 minutes.
7. ____ Apply the cold or ice directly on the skin to reduce swelling and bleeding.
8. ____ Elastic bandages can be applied too tightly.

Check (✓) the appropriate actions to relieve leg muscle cramps.

1. ____ Pinching the upper lip hard
2. ____ Drinking water (not saltwater)
3. ____ Taking salt tablets
4. ____ Gently stretching the affected muscle
5. ____ Applying ice to the cramped muscle

11

Medical Emergencies

■ Heart Attack ■ Stroke ■ Diabetic Emergencies ■
■ Epilepsy ■ Asthma ■

Heart Attack

A heart attack occurs when the blood supply to a part of the heart muscle is severely reduced or stopped because of an obstruction in one of the coronary arteries (these supply the heart with its blood). A buildup of fatty deposits along the coronary artery's inner wall is one reason for blood obstruction. The blood supply can also be reduced when the artery goes into a spasm.

Signs and Symptoms

Heart attacks are difficult to determine. Because medical care at the onset of a heart attack is vital to survival and the quality of recovery, the rule to follow is that if you suspect a heart attack for any reason, seek medical attention at once rather than delaying.

The American Heart Association lists these as possible signs and symptoms of a heart attack:

■ Uncomfortable pressure, fullness, squeezing or pain in the center of the chest lasting two minutes or longer. It may come and go.
■ Pain may spread to either shoulder, the neck, the lower jaw, or either arm.
■ Any or all of the following: weakness, dizziness, sweating, nausea, or shortness of breath.

Not all of these warning signs occur in every heart attack. Many victims will deny that they might be having a heart attack. If you see some of these signs, however, don't wait to seek medical attention. Time loss can seriously increase the risk of major damage. Get help immediately!

First Aid

The American Heart Association identifies these proper actions in case of a heart attack:

■ Find out which hospitals have 24-hour emergency cardiac care.
■ If chest discomfort lasts two minutes or more, call the emergency medical services.
■ If you can get to a hospital faster by going yourself and not waiting for an ambulance, drive the victim there.

Source: American Heart Association.

■ If you are with someone experiencing the signs and symptoms of a heart attack—and the warning signs last two minutes or longer—act immediately.
■ Expect a denial. It is normal for someone with chest discomfort to deny the possibility of something as serious as a heart attack. But don't take no for an answer. Insist on taking prompt action.
■ Call the emergency medical service or get to the nearest hospital emergency room offering 24-hour emergency cardiac care.
■ If necessary and if you are properly trained, give CPR.

Knowing these things, you should also:

■ Help the victim to the least painful position—usually sitting with legs up and bent at the knees. Loosen clothing around the neck and midriff. Be calm and reassuring.
■ Determine if the victim is *known* to have coronary heart disease and is using nitroglycerin. If so, use it. Nitroglycerin in tablets or spray under the tongue or in ointment placed on the skin may relieve chest pain. Nitroglycerin dilates the coronary artieries, which increases blood flow to the heart muscle; and it lowers the blood pressure and dilates the veins, which decreases the work of the heart and the heart muscle's need for oxygen.
Caution: Since nitroglycerin lowers blood pressure, the victim should be sitting or lying when taking it. Nitroglycerin may normally be repeated for a total of 3 tablets in 10 minutes if the first dose does not relieve the pain. However, a first aider may not know whether the victim has already taken some nitroglycerin. Also, nitroglycerin is prescribed in different strengths so that while 3 tablets of one strength may be a mild dose, 3 tablets of another strength may be a high dose. First aiders should be very cautious when administering nitroglycerin.
■ If victim is unconscious, check the ABCs and start CPR if needed.

Stroke*

A stroke is also known as a **cerebrovascular accident (CVA).** A stroke occurs when a blood vessel that is bringing oxygen and nutrients to the brain bursts or becomes clogged by a blood clot, preventing part of the brain from receiving the flow of blood it needs. Stroke is the third largest cause of death in America. It is also a major cause of disability.

Signs and Symptoms

Signs and symptoms of a stroke depend on the area of the brain involved:

- Sudden weakness or numbness of the face, arm and leg on one side of the body
- Loss of speech, or trouble talking or understanding speech
- Dimness or loss of vision, particularly in only one eye; unequal pupils
- Unexplained dizziness, unsteadiness or sudden falls
- Sudden severe headache
- Loss of bladder and/or bowel control

About 10% of strokes are preceded by "little strokes" (**transient ischemic attacks,** or TIAs). TIAs are extremely important warning signs for stroke. TIA symptoms are very similar to those of a full-fledged stroke. Do *not* ignore TIAs; get medical attention immediately.

First Aid

- Check and monitor the victim's breathing and pulse. Provide rescue breathing and/or cardiopulmonary resuscitation (CPR) if needed.
- If the victim is semiconscious or unconscious, place him or her on one side, preferably with the paralyzed side down. This position frees the victim's useful extremities. Cushion the paralyzed side. Positioning on the side permits secretions and vomit to drain into the cheek or out the mouth rather than the throat.
- Keep the victim in a semiprone position, preferably with the upper body and head slightly elevated to allow for less blood pressure on the brain.
- Remove dentures and any mucus and food from the mouth in a swabbing motion with a piece of cloth wrapped around a finger.
- Do *not* give any liquids—the throat may be paralyzed, which restricts swallowing.
- If an eye has been affected, consider protecting the eye by closing the lid and taping the eyelid down to prevent drying, which can result in vision loss.
- Provide calm reassurance to the victim.

Source: American Heart Association

Diabetic Emergencies*

Diabetes is the inability of the body to appropriately metabolize carbohydrates. The pancreas fails to produce enough of a hormone called insulin. The function of insulin is to take sugar from the blood and carry it into the cells to be used. When excess sugar remains in the blood, the body cells must rely on fat as fuel. Since blood sugar is a major body fuel, when it cannot be used, diabetes develops.

When the blood sugar level becomes too high because of too little insulin in the blood, diabetic coma, or **ketoacidosis**, may occur. Meanwhile, the cells, deprived of sugar, begin to use fats for fuel. Use of fat results in the production of acids and ketones as wastes. The ketones give the victims' breath a fruity odor.

The opposite condition, insulin shock, can result when a person with diabetes has taken too much insulin or has not eaten. The blood sugar level drops dangerously low, and the victim becomes weak and disoriented, or unconscious.

Both of these conditions can be fatal unless something is done to reverse them. See page 151 for a description of symptoms and first aid for diabetic emergencies.

Epilepsy**

Types of Seizures

Epileptic seizures may be convulsive or nonconvulsive in nature, depending on where in the brain the malfunction takes place and on how much of the total brain area is involved.

Convulsive seizures are the ones that most people generally think of when they hear the word "epilepsy." In this type of seizure the person undergoes convulsions that usually last from two to five minutes, with complete loss of consciousness and muscle spasm.

Nonconvulsive seizures may take the form of a blank stare lasting only a few seconds, an involuntary movement of an arm or leg, or a period of automatic movement in which awareness of one's surroundings is blurred or completely absent.

Since these seizure types are so different, they require different kinds of action from a first aider, and some require no action at all. Table 11.2 describes seizures in detail and how to handle each type.

First Aid

An uncomplicated convulsive seizure due to epilepsy is not a medical emergency, even though it looks like

Source: American Diabetes Association; reprinted with permission.
**Source: Epilepsy Foundation of America; reprinted with permission.*

In an emergency
THINK DIABETES!

LOW Blood Sugar
(Insulin reaction or Hypoglycemia)

Symptoms
Sudden Onset
Staggering, poor coordination
Anger, bad temper
Pale color
Confusion, disorientation
Sudden hunger
Sweating
Eventual stupor or
unconsciousness

Action to take:

Provide sugar! If the person can swallow without choking, offer any food or drink containing sugar, such as soft drinks, fruit juice, or candy. Do not use diet drinks when blood sugar is low.

If the person does not respond in 10 to 15 minutes, take him/her to the hospital.

HIGH Blood Sugar
(Hyperglycemia or Acidosis)

Symptoms
Gradual Onset
Drowsiness
Extreme thirst
Very frequent urination
Flushed skin
Vomiting
Fruity or wine-like breath odor
Heavy breathing
Eventual stupor or
unconsciousness

Action to take:

Take this person to the hospital. If you are uncertain whether the person is suffering from high or low blood sugar, give some sugar-containing food or drink. If there is no response in 10-15 minutes, this person needs immediate medical attention.

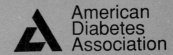

American Diabetes Association

Warning: A diabetic emergency may resemble alcohol or drug intoxication. Know the symptoms of low and high blood sugar. **THINK DIABETES!**

---

one. After a few minutes it stops naturally, without ill effects. The average victim is able to resume normal activity after a rest period and may need little or no assistance in getting home.

However, several medical conditions other than epilepsy can cause seizures. These require immediate medical attention and include:

encephalitis	pregnancy
meningitis	hypoglycemia
heat stroke	high fever
poisoning	head injury

The following guidelines are designed to help people with epilepsy avoid unnecessary and expensive trips to the emergency room and to help you decide whether or not to call an ambulance when someone has a convulsive seizure. Reasons to call the EMS system include:

- A seizure that lasts more than five minutes.
- There is no "epilepsy" or "seizure disorder" identification.
- Slow recovery, a second seizure, or difficult breathing afterwards.

- Pregnancy or other medical condition identification.
- Any signs of injury or illnesses.

The Epilepsy Foundation of America lists these first aid procedures for seizures (convulsions, generalized tonic-clonic, grand mal seizures):

1. Cushion the victim's head
2. Loosen the victim's tight neckwear
3. Turn the victim onto side
4. Look for a medic alert tag (bracelet or necklace)
5. As seizure ends, offer your help. Most seizures in people with epilepsy are not medical emergencies. They end after a minute or two without harm and usually do not require medical attention.

Precautions in caring for a seizure victim:

- Do *not* give anything to eat or drink.
- Do *not* hold the victim down.
- Do *not* put anything between the victim's teeth during the seizure.
- Do *not* throw any liquid on the victim's face or into his or her mouth.

TABLE 11-2 Seizure: Recognition and First Aid

Seizure Type	What It Looks Like	What it is Not	What To Do	What Not To Do
Generalized Tonic-Clonic (Also called grand mal)	Sudden cry, fall, rigidity, followed by muscle jerks, shallow breathing or temporarily suspended breathing, bluish skin, possible loss of bladder or bowel control, usually lasts a couple of minutes. Normal breathing then starts again. There may be some confusion and/or fatigue, followed by return to full consciousness.	Heart attack Stroke	Look for medical identification. Protect from nearby hazards. Loosen tie or shirt collars. Protect head from injury. Turn on side to keep airway clear. Reassure when consciousness returns. If single seizure lasted less than 5 minutes, ask if hospital evaluation wanted. If multiple seizures, or if one seizure lasts longer than 5 minutes, call an ambulance. If person is pregnant, injured or diabetic, call for aid at once.	Don't put any hard implement in the mouth. Don't try to hold tongue. It can't be swallowed. Don't try to give liquids during or just after seizure. Don't use artificial respiration unless breathing is absent after muscle jerks subside, or unless water has been inhaled. Don't restrain.
Absence (Also called petit mal)	A blank stare, lasting only a few seconds, most common in children. May be accompanied by rapid blinking, some chewing movements of the mouth. Child is unaware of what's going on during the seizure, but quickly returns to full awareness once it has stopped. May result in learning difficulties if not recognized and treated.	Daydreaming Lack of attention Deliberate ignoring of adult instructions	No first aid necessary, but if this is the first observation of the seizure(s), medical evaluation should be recommended.	
Simple Partial	Jerking may begin in one area of the body, arm, leg, or face. Can't be stopped, but patient stays awake and aware. Jerking may proceed from one area of the body to another, and sometimes spreads to become a convulsive seizure. Partial sensory seizures may not be obvious to an onlooker. Patient experiences a distorted environment. May see or hear things that aren't there, may feel unexplained fear, sadness, anger, or joy. May have nausea, experience odd smells, and have a generally "funny" feeling in the stomach.	Acting out, bizarre behavior Hysteria Mental Illness Psychosomatic illness Parapsychological or mystical experience	No first aid necessary unless seizure becomes convulsive, then first aid as above. No action needed other than reassurance and emotional support. Medical evaluation should be recommended.	
Complex Partial (Also called psychomotor or temporal lobe)	Usually starts with blank stare, followed by chewing, followed by random activity. Person appears unaware of surroundings, may seem dazed and mumble. Unresponsive. Actions clumsy, not directed. May pick at clothing, pick up objects, try to take clothes off. May run, appear to be afraid. May struggle or flail at restraint. Once pattern established, same set of actions usually occur with each seizure. Lasts a few	Drunkenness Intoxication on drugs Mental Illness Disorderly conduct	Speak calmly and reassuringly to patient and others. Guide gently away from obvious hazards. Stay with person until completely aware of environment. Offer to help getting home.	Don't grab hold unless sudden danger (such as a cliff edge or an approaching car) threatens. Don't try to restrain. Don't shout. Don't expect verbal instructions to be obeyed.

TABLE 11-2 Seizure: Recognition and First Aid (continued)

Seizure Type	What It Looks Like	What it is Not	What To Do	What Not To Do
Complex Partial Cont.	minutes, but post-seizure confusion can last substantially longer. No memory of what happened during seizure period.			
Atonic Seizures (Also called drop attacks)	A child or adult suddenly collapses and falls. After 10 seconds to a minute he recovers, regains consciousness, and can stand and walk again.	Clumsiness Normal childhood "stage" In a child, lack of good walking skills In an adult, drunkenness, accute illness	No first aid needed (unless he hurt himself as he fell), but the child should be given a thorough medical evaluation.	
Myoclonic Seizures	Sudden brief, massive muscle jerks that may involve the whole body or parts of body. May cause person to spill what they were holding or fall off a chair.	Clumsiness Poor coordination	No first aid needed, but should be given a thorough medical evaluation.	
Infantile Spasms	These are clusters of quick, sudden movements that start between 3 months and two years. If a child is sitting up, the head will fall forward, and the arms will flex forward. If lying down, the knees will be drawn up, with arms and head flexed forward as if the baby is reaching for support.	Normal movements of the baby Colic	No first aid, but doctor should be consulted.	

Source: © Epilepsy Foundation of America; reprinted with permission.

Asthma

Asthma results from a narrowing of the airway bronchial tubes, causing breathing difficulty, especially while exhaling. Wheezing is a whistling, high-pitched sound produced by air forced through a constricted airway. Not all wheezes involve asthma.

Signs and Symptoms

- Breathing difficulty while exhaling
- Wheezing or whistling sound
- Tense, frightened, nervous behavior
- Bluish skin color in severe attacks due to lack of oxygen
- Preference for sitting up (since it is easier to breathe).

First Aid

In most cases, the first aider can do little other than recognize asthma and, if needed, obtain medical assistance. Provide the following for the victim:

- Comfort and reassure victim since emotional stress can make the condition worse.
- Many asthmatics carry tablets or inhalers that relax bronchial spasms. Help them in using these medicines.
- Help the victim into a comfortable breathing position that he or she chooses. The best position is usually sitting upright.
- Place the victim in a room that is as free as possible of common offenders (e.g., dust, feathers, animals). It should also be free of odors (e.g., tobacco smoke, paint).
- Keep conversations with asthmatics brief since they are struggling to breathe.
- Increase the drinking of water if possible.
- Seek medical attention, for:

  1. Severe, prolonged asthma attacks

  2. Reactions happening after an insect sting or contact with another source that produces an allergic reaction, which could progress to anaphylactic shock

  3. Failure to improve with medication

  4. Breathing that can barely be heard

  5. Increasing bluish skin color

  6. Pulse rate of more than 120 beats per minute

■ HEART ATTACK ■

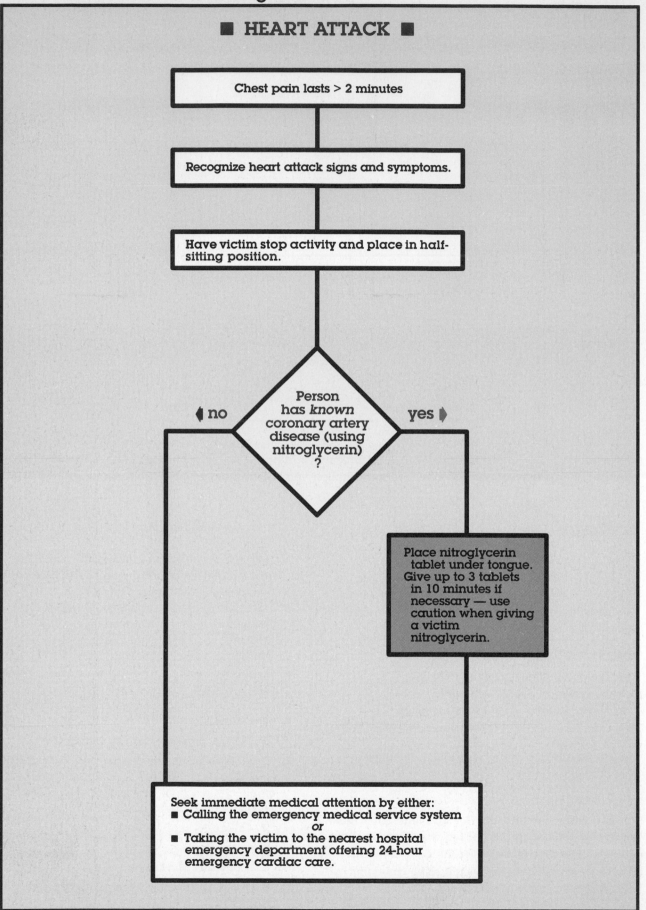

Chest pain lasts > 2 minutes

Recognize heart attack signs and symptoms.

Have victim stop activity and place in half-sitting position.

Person has *known* coronary artery disease (using nitroglycerin)?

◀ no   yes ▶

Place nitroglycerin tablet under tongue. Give up to 3 tablets in 10 minutes if necessary — use caution when giving a victim nitroglycerin.

Seek immediate medical attention by either:
■ Calling the emergency medical service system
or
■ Taking the victim to the nearest hospital emergency department offering 24-hour emergency cardiac care.

■ STROKE ■

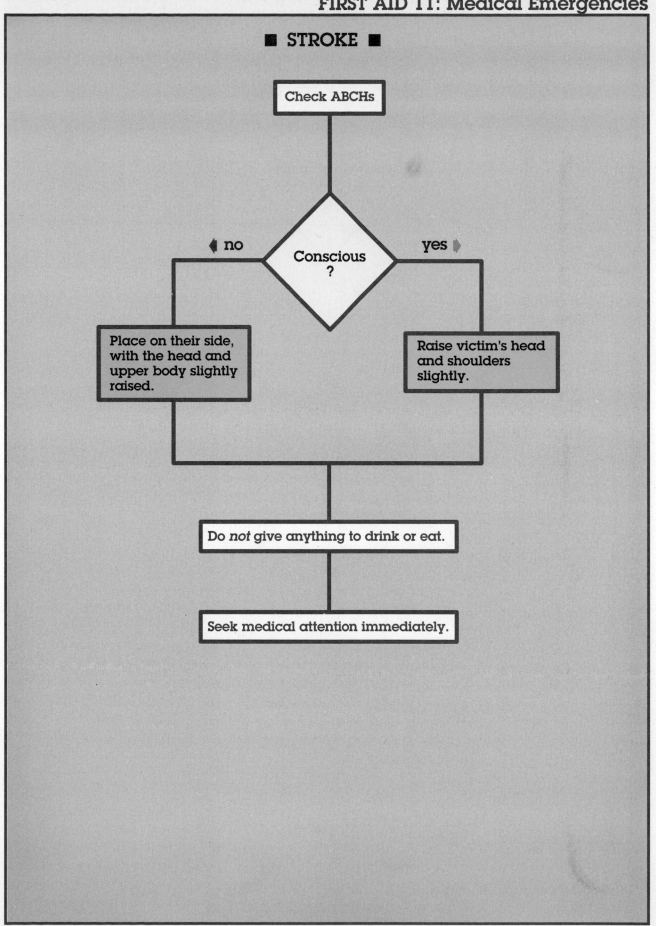

Check ABCHs

Conscious?

no — Place on their side, with the head and upper body slightly raised.

yes — Raise victim's head and shoulders slightly.

Do *not* give anything to drink or eat.

Seek medical attention immediately.

■ DIABETIC EMERGENCIES ■

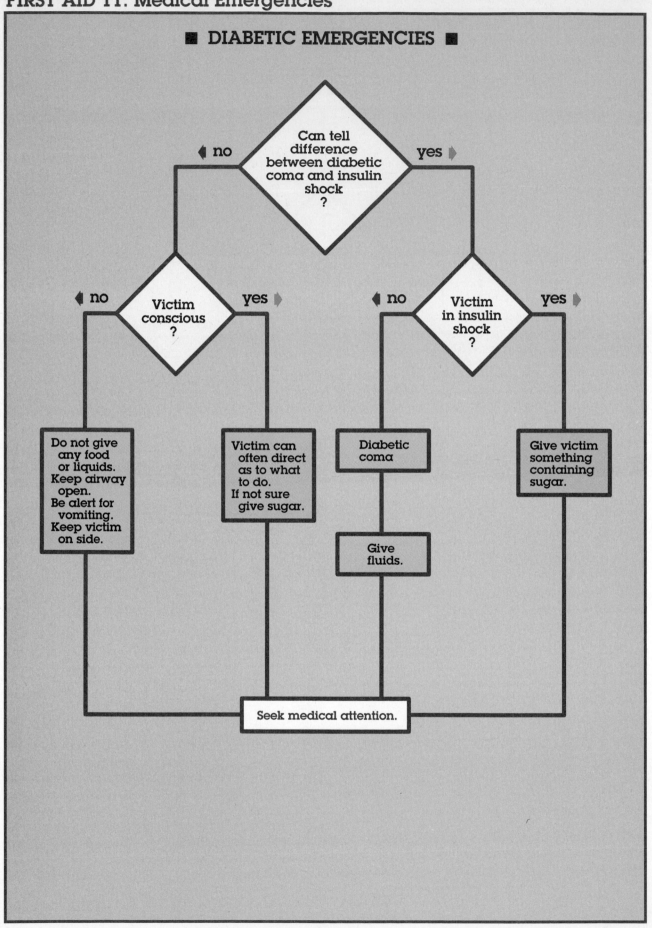

■ SEIZURES ■

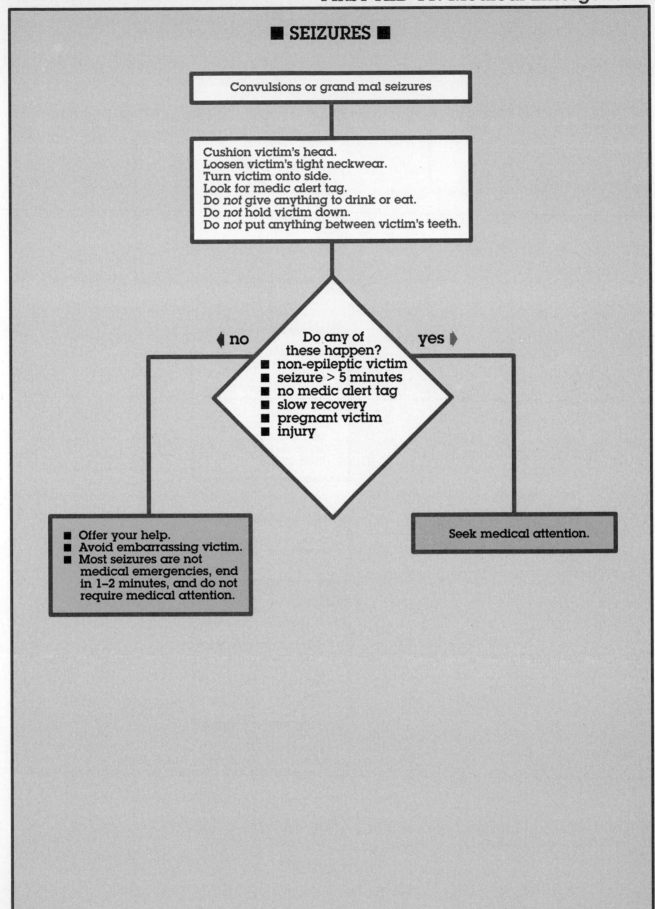

Convulsions or grand mal seizures

Cushion victim's head.
Loosen victim's tight neckwear.
Turn victim onto side.
Look for medic alert tag.
Do *not* give anything to drink or eat.
Do *not* hold victim down.
Do *not* put anything between victim's teeth.

Do any of these happen?
- non-epileptic victim
- seizure > 5 minutes
- no medic alert tag
- slow recovery
- pregnant victim
- injury

◀ no   yes ▶

- Offer your help.
- Avoid embarrassing victim.
- Most seizures are not medical emergencies, end in 1–2 minutes, and do not require medical attention.

Seek medical attention.

■ ASTHMA ■

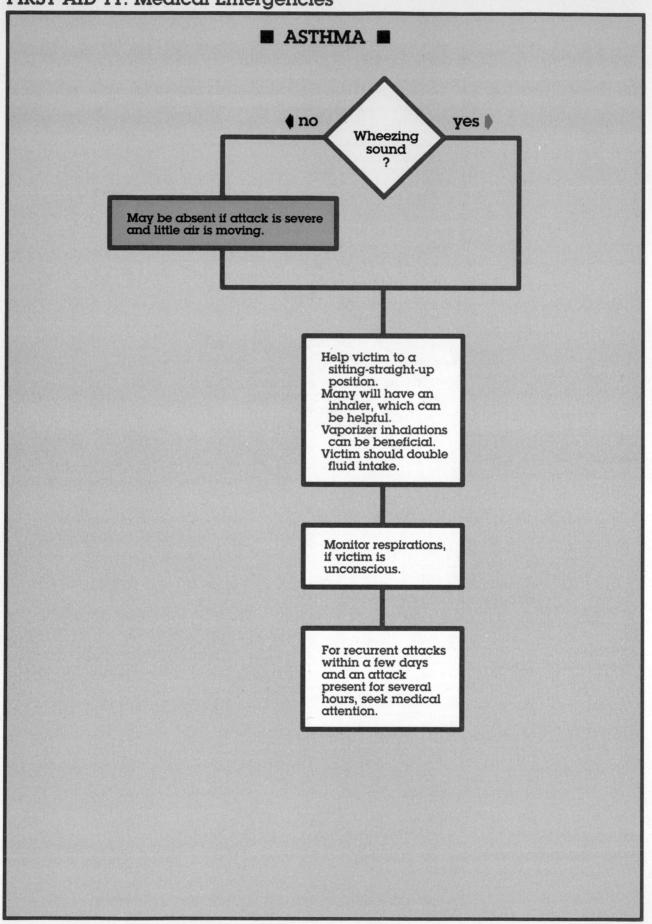

Wheezing sound ?

◄ no

yes ▶

May be absent if attack is severe and little air is moving.

Help victim to a sitting-straight-up position.
Many will have an inhaler, which can be helpful.
Vaporizer inhalations can be beneficial.
Victim should double fluid intake.

Monitor respirations, if victim is unconscious.

For recurrent attacks within a few days and an attack present for several hours, seek medical attention.

■ ACTIVITY 1 ■
Heart Attack

Check the appropriate sign(s) and symptom(s).

A person having a heart attack may have which of the following signs and symptoms?

1. _____ Complaint of a squeezing chest pain

2. _____ Leg cramping

3. _____ Excessive sweating

4. _____ Appearance of weakness and complaint of dizziness

5. _____ Fruity breath odor

6. _____ Seizure

Mark each action yes (Y) or no (N).

What should you do if a co-worker complains about chest pain, making you suspect a heart attack?

1. _____ Quickly call for an ambulance.

2. _____ Help the victim move and stretch his arms.

3. _____ Help the victim to a lying down position.

4. _____ If the heart stops, a trained person should give CPR.

5. _____ Place the victim in a semisitting position.

■ ACTIVITY 2 ■
Stroke

Mark each sign or symptom yes (Y) or no (N).

Which of the following may indicate a stroke has occurred?

1. _____ A sudden, severe headache

2. _____ The pupil of one eye is larger than the pupil of the other eye

3. _____ Chest pain and nausea complaints

4. _____ No feeling on one side of the body

5. _____ Swelling in the left arm and leg

6. _____ Speech affected

Mark each action yes (Y) or no (N).

For a suspected stroke, which of the following should you do?

1. _____ Relieve the victim's anxieties by being calmly reassuring.

2. _____ Give a glass of water to drink.

3. _____ Keep head propped up.

4. _____ If unconscious, place the victim on the paralyzed side.

Write the appropriate letter in each space below to specify whether the signs and symptoms described indicate (A) a heart attack or (B) a stroke.

1. _____ Sudden numbness of the face

2. _____ Sweating, nausea, and vomiting

3. _____ Chest pain and feelings of nausea

4. _____ Unequal size of pupils of the eyes

5. _____ Partial paralysis of the body

■ ACTIVITY 3 ■
Diabetic Emergencies

Mark each action yes (Y) or no (N).

Which of the following actions should you take when a diabetic emergency occurs?

1. ____ Look for a medic alert tag on the person's wrist or neck.

2. ____ Give a conscious diabetic several glasses of a diet drink.

3. ____ Wait 30 minutes to see if the person's condition improves.

4. ____ Give a conscious diabetic anything containing sugar if there is any doubt about which diabetic emergency is involved.

■ ACTIVITY 4 ■
Epilepsy

Mark each action yes (Y) or no (N).

Which of the following actions should you take when a convulsive seizure happens?

1. ____ Put a "bite stick" or other hard implement between victim's teeth.

2. ____ Hold the victim down.

3. ____ Give some water during or just after a seizure.

4. ____ Look for medical identification.

5. ____ Loosen tight clothing around neck (e.g., tie).

6. ____ Turn on side to prevent choking.

7. ____ Person in a seizure lasting longer than 10 minutes should be taken to emergency room.

8. ____ Take victim to emergency room if multiple seizures occur.

■ ACTIVITY 5 ■
Asthma

Mark the statements true (T) or false (F).

1. ____ In most asthma cases a first aider can do little except obtain medical assistance if needed.

2. ____ Don't give water because of possible choking.

3. ____ A vaporizer may be helpful.

4. ____ Inhaling nebulized medication can be effective.

5. ____ The best position for the victim is usually lying down on one side.

6. ____ Keep the victim talking since it keeps the air moving into the lungs.

12
First Aid Skills
■ Bandaging ■ Splinting ■

Dressings control bleeding and prevent contamination. Bandages hold dressings in place. Dressings come in many different forms. Sterile gauzes are most commonly used. When these cannot be found, nonsterile substances such as towels or handkerchiefs can be applied. Many different forms of bandages exist. Roller gauze, triangular, and cravat bandages make up the bandages most often used by first aiders. However, self-adhering and formfitting bandages have become popular especially with emergency medical technicians.

Bandages need not be textbook perfect as long as they hold the dressings in place. Care should be taken, however, so that bandages are not applied too tightly or too loosely. Too tightly applied bandages will restrict blood flow, and too loose bandages fail to hold the dressing in place. When extremities are bandaged,

the fingers and toes should be left exposed so that any color changes in them can be noted. Such changes may indicate impaired circulation. Pain, color change, numbness, and tingling are other signs of a too-tight bandage.

Methods of applying dressings and bandages vary greatly and differ according to the types used and the injured part to which they are applied. Because of the variety of good bandaging techniques, the examples shown on the following pages represent a consensus among first aid experts as to the appropriate methods.

These illustrations show suggested bandaging and splinting skills. This compilation represents the skills needed for first aid situations most likely to be encountered.

TABLE 12-1 Splinting Guide

Injured Part	Suggested splinting materials and methods
Spine	Long backboard, best applied by trained EMS personnel; immobilize and wait
Collarbone	Sling and swathe*
Ribs	Victim holds pillow over injury
Upper arm	Rigid** splint on outside; wrist sling and swathe*
Elbow	**Straight**: rigid** splint on inside of arm **Bent**: rigid** splint on inside of arm; wrist sling
Forearm/Wrist	Rigid** splint; sling and swathe*
Hand	Keep hand in position of function with a wadded cloth in palm; tie hand to rigid** splint; sling and swathe*
Finger(s)	Splint same as hand or tape finger to uninjured finger and apply sling
Pelvis/Hip	Long backboard, best applied by trained EMS personnel
Thigh	Tie legs together or use 2 long boards or traction splint applied by trained EMS personnel
Knee	**Straight**: rigid** splint behind leg **Bent**: rigid** splint on outside of leg
Lower leg	Rigid** splints on sides or tie legs together
Foot/ankle	Pillow splint
Toe	Tape toe to uninjured toe

KEY: **Swathe*** = binder (usually a cravat bandage) tied around body to hold arm against body to decrease movement; used on most upper extremity fractures.

Rigid* = must be long enough to include adjacent joints; examples include padded boards, 40 pages of folded newspapers, or cardboard.

MAKING A CRAVAT

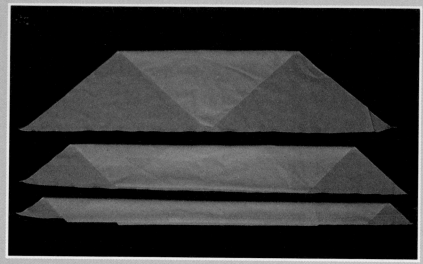

Cravat bandage for head, ears, or eyes

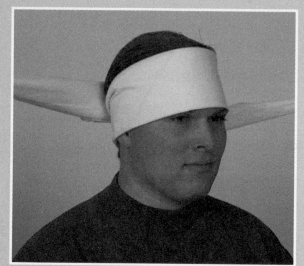

1.

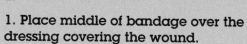

2.

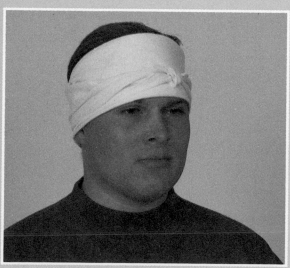

3.

1. Place middle of bandage over the dressing covering the wound.

2. Cross the two ends snugly over each other.

3. Bring the ends back around to where the dressing is and tie the ends in a knot.

Cravat bandage for arm or leg

Cravat bandage for elbow or knee

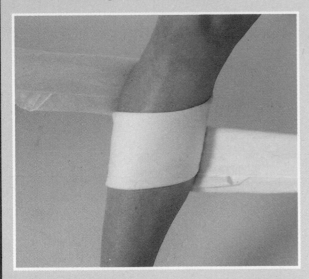

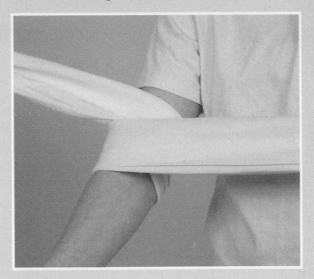

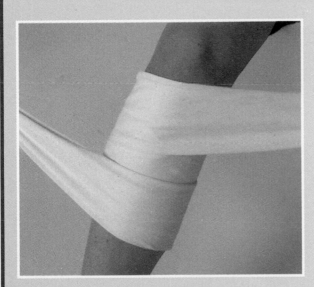

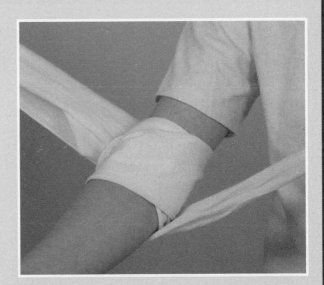

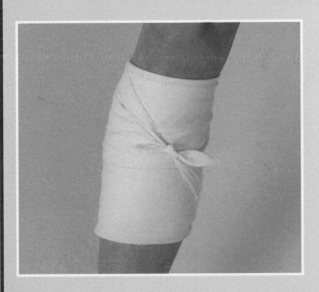

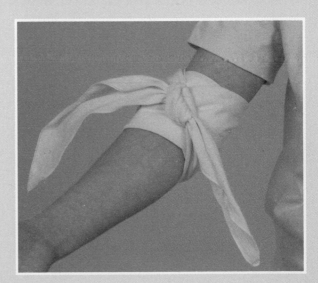

Roller bandage for hand

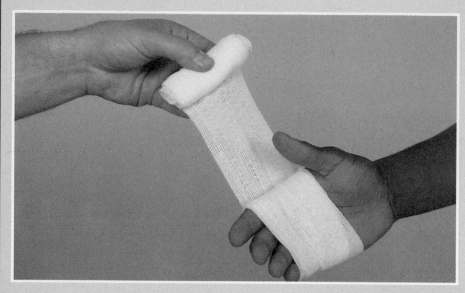

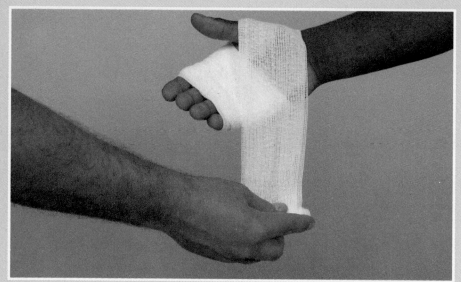

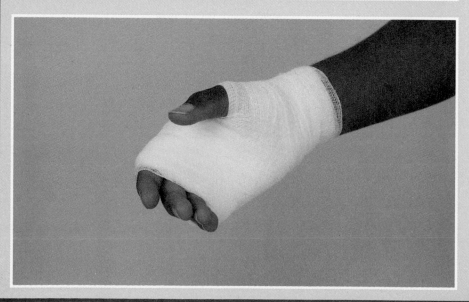

Roller bandage for elbow or knee

Roller bandage for ankle

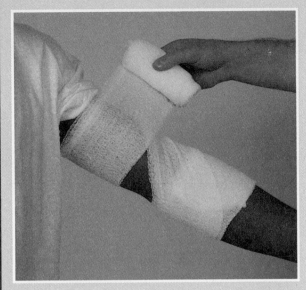

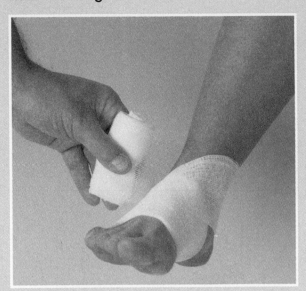

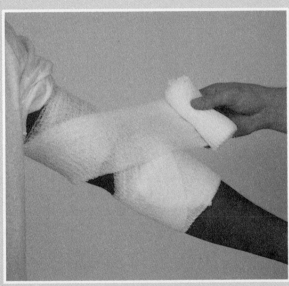

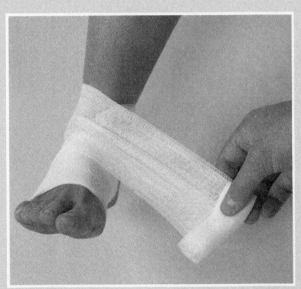

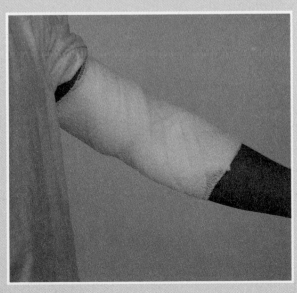

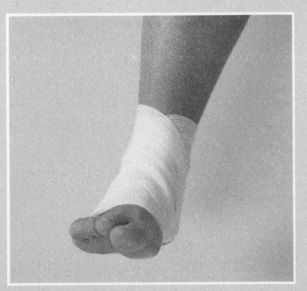

ARM SLING: COLLARBONE, SHOULDER   UPPER ARM (HUMERUS)

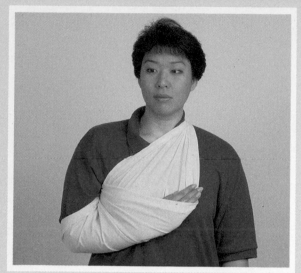

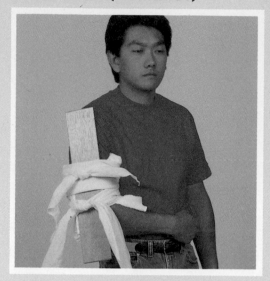

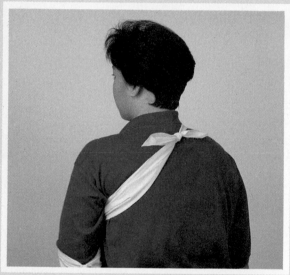

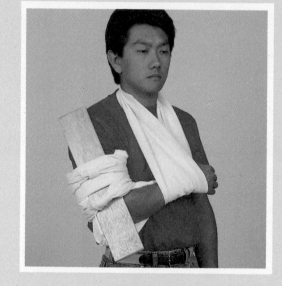

ARM SLING AND SWATHE (BINDER)

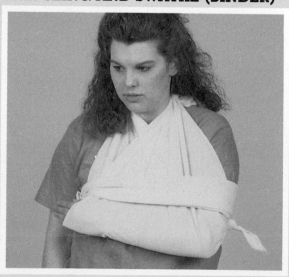

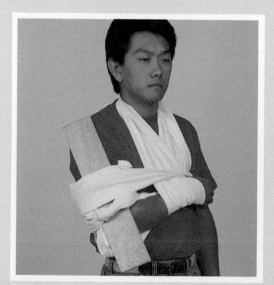

**FOREARM
(RADIUS/ULNA)**

**FINGERS AND HAND
(POSITION OF FUNCTION)**

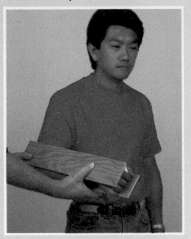

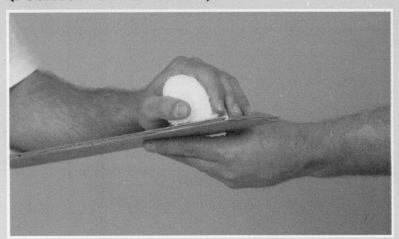

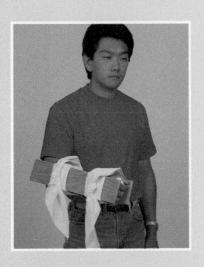

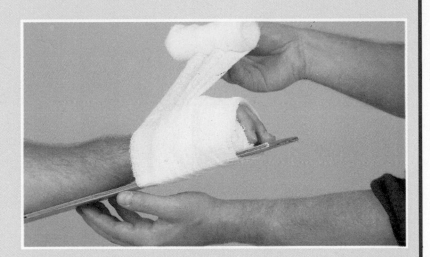

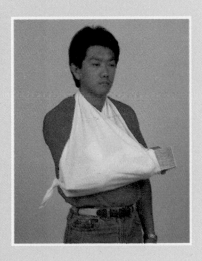

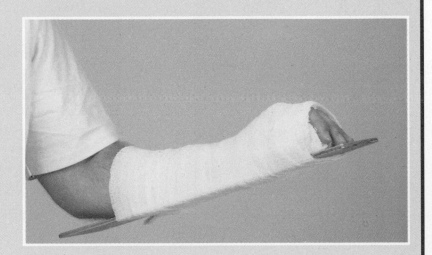

ELBOW IN BENT POSITION

ELBOW IN STRAIGHT POSITION

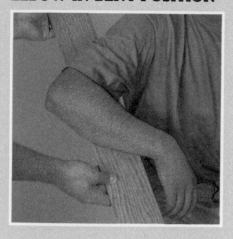

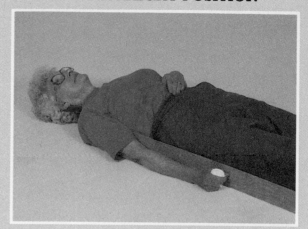

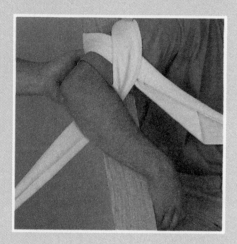

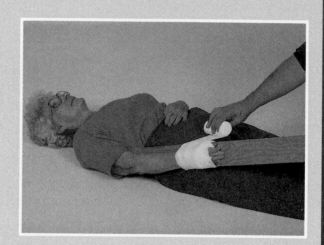

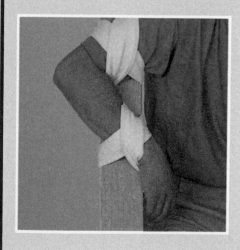

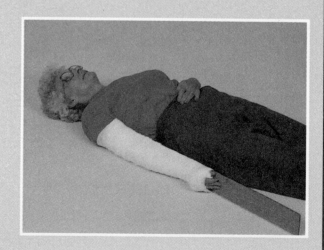

SPLINTING THE LOWER LEG (TIBIA/FIBULA)

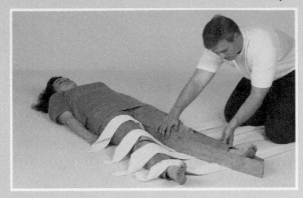

1.

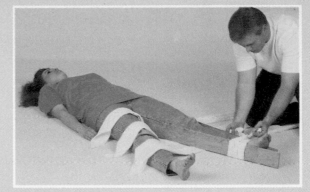

2.

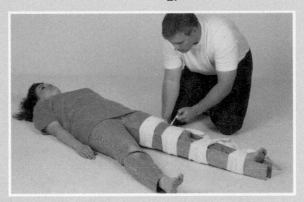

3.

THIGH (FEMUR)

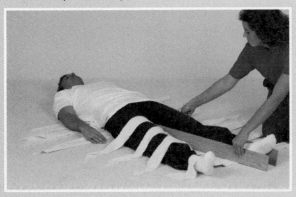

1.

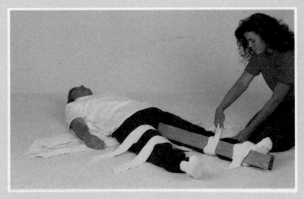

2.

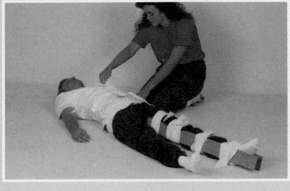

3.

SKILL SCAN: Splinting—Lower Extremities

ANKLE/FOOT

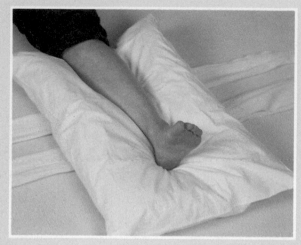

1.

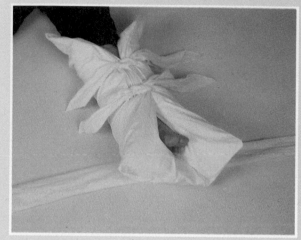

2.

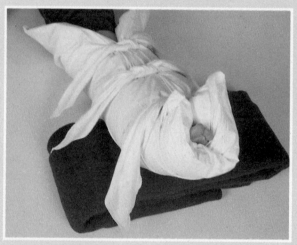

3.

SPLINTING—SELF-SPLINT

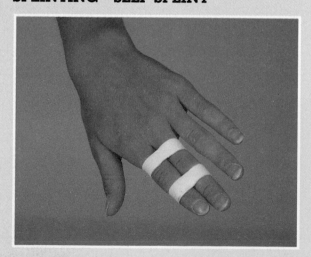

Fingers/toes

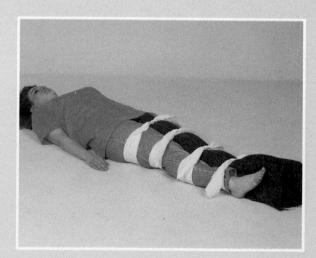

Leg

SKILL SCAN: Splinting—Knee

KNEE IN BENT POSITION

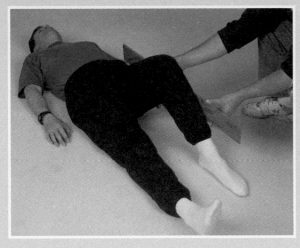

1.

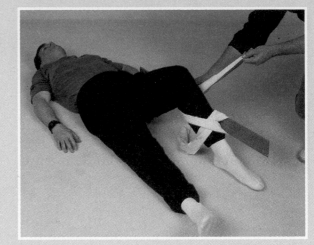

2.

KNEE IN STRAIGHT POSITION

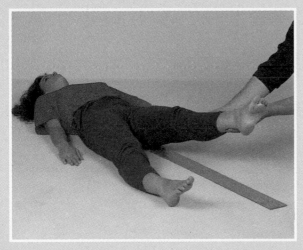

1.

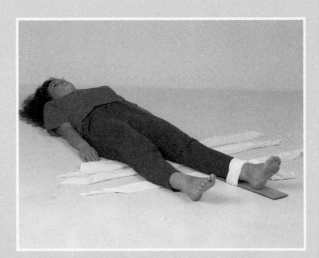

2.

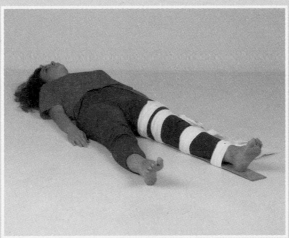

3.

SKILL SCAN: Splinting—Knee

13

Moving and Rescuing Victims

■ Emergency Moves ■ Nonemergency Moves ■
■ Water Rescue ■

In general, a victim should not be moved until he or she is ready for transportation to a hospital, if required. All necessary first aid should be provided first. A victim should be moved only if there is an immediate danger, that is:

■ There is a fire or danger of fire.
■ Explosives or other hazardous materials are involved.
■ It is impossible to protect the accident scene.
■ It is impossible to gain access to other victims in a vehicle who need life-saving care.

Note that a cardiac arrest victim would typically be moved unless he or she were on the ground or floor because cardiopulmonary resuscitation must be performed on a firm surface.

If it is necessary to move a victim, the speed of movement depends on the reason for moving, for example:

■ **Emergency move.** If there is a fire, pull the victim away from the area as quickly as possible.
■ **Nonemergency move.** If the victim needs to be moved to gain access to others in a vehicle, give due consideration to injuries before and during movement.

Emergency Moves

The major danger in moving a victim quickly is the possibility of aggravating spine injury. In an emergency, every effort should be made to pull the victim in the direction of the long axis of the body to provide as much protection to the spine as possible. If victims are on the floor or ground, you can drag them away from the scene by tugging on their clothing in the neck and shoulder area. It may be easier to pull a victim onto a blanket and then drag the blanket away from the scene. Such moves are emergency moves only. They do not adequately protect the spine from further injury.

Nonemergency Moves

All injured parts should be immobilized before moving and then protected during the moving. To protect yourself, you should use the following principles in all nonemergency moves:

■ Keep in mind physical capabilities and limitations and do not try to handle too heavy a load. When in doubt, seek help.
■ Keep yourself balanced when carrying out the move.
■ Maintain a firm footing.
■ Maintain a constant and firm grip.
■ Lift and lower by bending your legs and not your back—keep your back as straight as possible at all times; bend knees and lift with one foot ahead of the other.
■ When holding or transporting, keep your back straight and rely on shoulder and leg muscles; tighten muscles of your abdomen and buttocks.
■ When performing a task that requires pulling, keep your back straight and pull, using your arms and shoulders.
■ Carry out all tasks slowly, smoothly, and in unison with your partner.
■ Move your body gradually; avoid twisting and jerking when conducting the various victim-handling tasks.
■ When handling a victim, try to keep your arms as close as possible to the body in order to maintain balance.
■ Do not keep your muscles contracted for a long period of time.

Transporting an injured victim by stretcher is safer and more comfortable for the victim than by other methods. It is also easier for the rescuers. A common type of stretcher is the army, or canvas stretcher. It consists of two poles with canvas attached. Stretchers can be improvised using various materials, for example: a house door removed from its hinges, a ladder, or any two strong poles and material (e.g., blanket, canvas). If strong material is available but there is nothing for poles, you can place the victim in the center

CARRIES

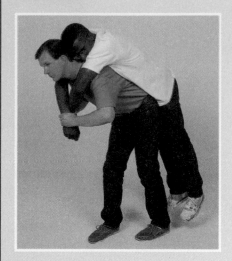

Pack-strap carry

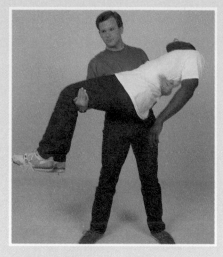

Cradle carry

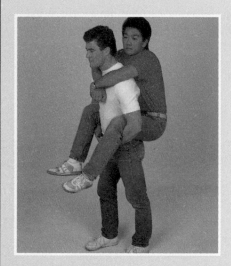

Piggyback carry

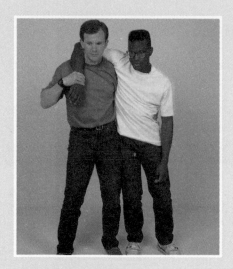

One-person assist

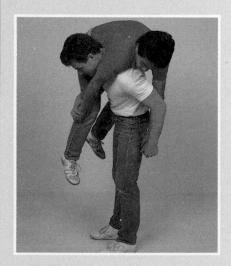

Fireman's carry

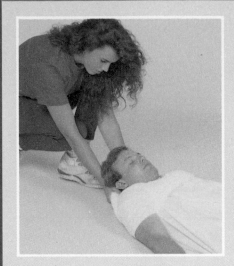

Sling drag

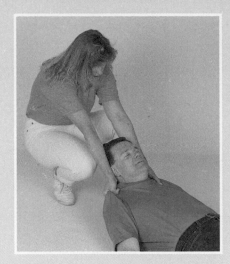

Clothing drag

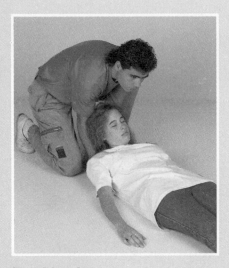

Shoulder drag

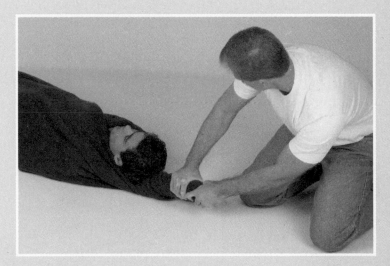

Blanket drag

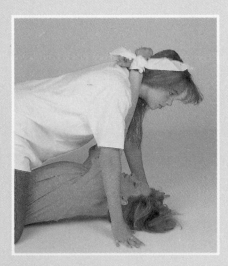

Fireman's drag

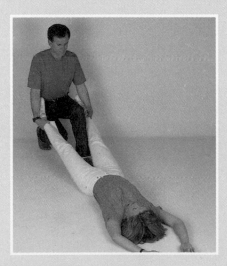

Ankle drag

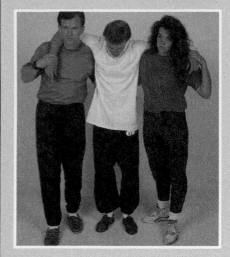

Two-person assist

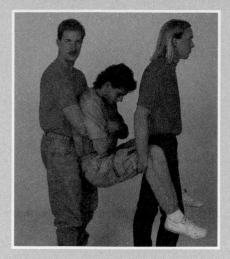

Extremity carry

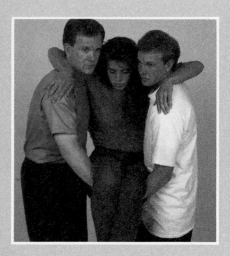

Two-handed seat carry

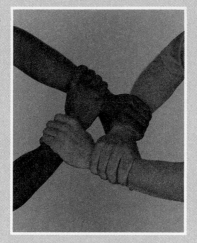

Four-handed grip

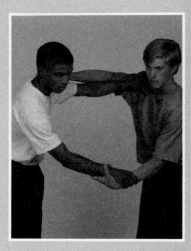

Two-handed grip

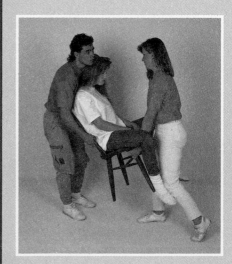

Chair carry

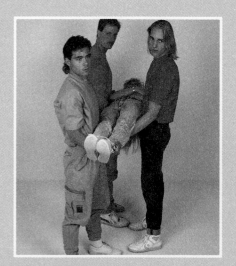

Hammock carry

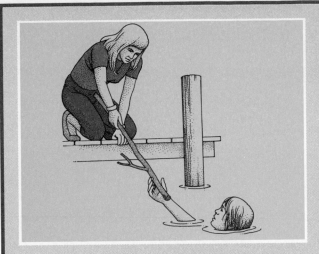

1. Reach the person from shore.

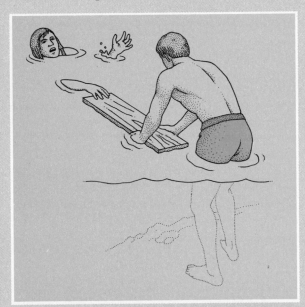

2. If you cannot reach the person from shore, wade closer.

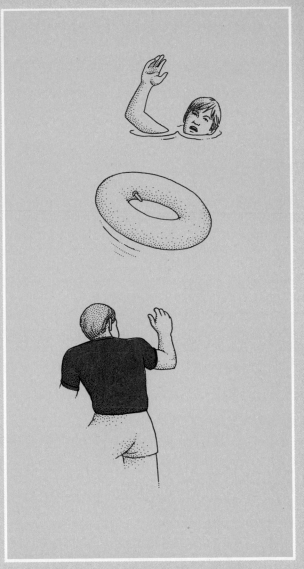

3. If an object that floats is available, throw it to the person.

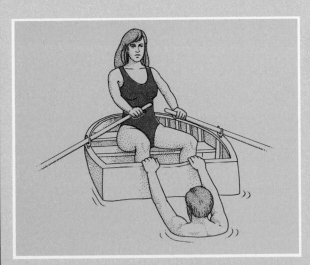

4. Use a boat if one is available.

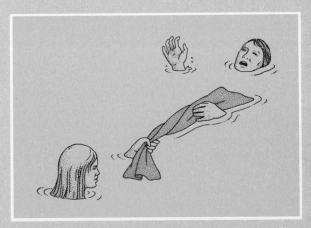

5. If you must swim to the person, use a towel or board for him or her to hold onto. Do not let the person grab you.

of the material, tightly roll the sides snug against the victim, and use them for handholds to be carried by four or more people. Test the improvised stretcher before using.

Many improvised stretchers are not rigid enough to be used for victims needing CPR or those with potential spinal injuries. Whenever possible, moving seriously injured or ill victims should be left to trained EMS personnel.

Water Rescue

About 7,000 Americans die each year from drowning, making it the third leading cause of accidental death. Drowning statistics do not reflect the whole problem. An estimated 70,000 people are near-drowning victims each year. Even this figure does not give the entire picture because in many instances the victim recovers and the incident is not reported.

Since drowning situations seem to happen all the time, especially during the summer months, all adults and teenagers should be familiar with the basic rescue techniques available to poor swimmers or nonswimmers.

Reach-Throw-Row-Go

Reach-throw-row-go identifies the priority list for attempting a rescue.

Reach

The first and simplest rescue technique is the reach. This method is easily mastered, but it requires the ability to judge distance accurately and a lightweight pole, ladder, long stick, or any object that can be extended to the victim.

Once you have your "reacher," secure your footing. Also have a bystander grab your belt or pants for stability. Make sure you are secure before reaching down to assist the victim. Keep talking; this not only calms the victim, it helps you think through each step.

Throw

Throwing is another elementary rescue. It provides a maximum range of about fifty feet for the average untrained rescuer. You can throw anything that floats—objects such as empty fuel or paint cans, plastic containers, life jackets or floating cushions, short pieces of wood—whatever is available. If there is rope handy, tie it to the object to be thrown because you can retrieve it in case you miss.

Row

If the victim is beyond reach and you can find a nearby sailboard, boogie board, rowboat, canoe, or an outboard craft that can be started, you may attempt this form of rescue. Using these crafts requires skill only acquired through practice. In a life-or-death situation, however, even the inept use of these craft will be safer and faster than a swimming rescue. There is an element of danger for the rescuer that should be considered.

Craft powered by hand, paddle, or oar may be slower, but they are safer than a motor-driven craft with which you are unfamiliar. Inexperienced hands on a throttle are more dangerous than inexperienced hands on an oar.

If rowing out to a victim, align with an object on the shoreline and in line with the victim. Fix this in your memory. Since you must row facing the opposite direction, you will need to turn your head every five or so strokes to check on the victim and your position.

Upon reaching the victim, never attempt to pull the victim in over the sides of a boat but over the stern or rear end. The former method has been the cause of countless double drownings.

Go

If the previous "reach-throw-row" priorities are impossible to do, you must make an assessment, weighing the potential risk to yourself versus the reward to the victim. Entering even calm water to make a swimming rescue is difficult and hazardous. It takes skill, training, and excellent physical condition. All too frequently a would-be rescuer becomes a victim as well.

Underwater Duration

In 1986, two-year-old Michelle Funk of Salt Lake City, Utah, made a full recovery after spending 66 minutes underwater. The toddler fell into a swollen creek near her home while playing. When she was eventually discovered, rescue workers found she had no pulse or heartbeat. Her life was saved by the first successful bypass machine to warm blood, which had dropped to 66°F. Doctors at the hospital described the time she had spent underwater as the "longest documented submergence with an intact neurological outcome."

The record for voluntarily staying underwater is 13 minutes 42.5 seconds by Robert Foster, aged 32, of Richmond, California, who stayed under 10 feet of water in a swimming pool in San Rafael, California on March 15, 1959. He hyperventilated with oxygen for 30 minutes before his descent. *It must be stressed that record-breaking of this kind is extremely dangerous.*

—Guinness Book of World Records

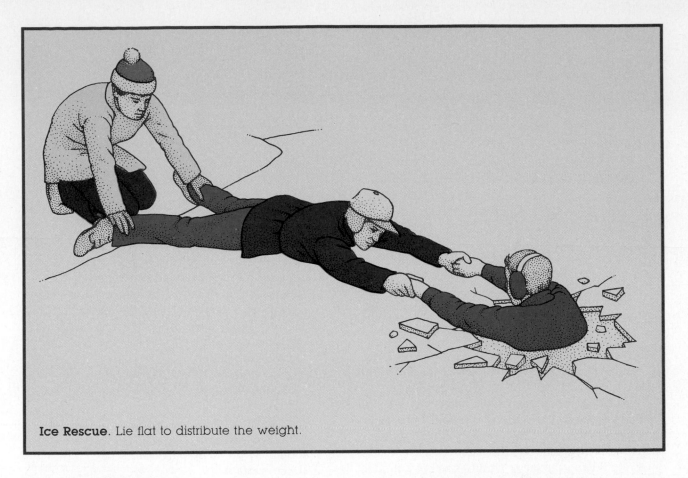

Ice Rescue. Lie flat to distribute the weight.

After the Rescue

Once the victim is out of the water, protect yourself and the victim against the cold. Get into dry clothing as soon as possible. Be prepared to administer mouth-to-mouth or CPR resuscitation. All rescued victims should be seen by a physician and hospitalized because victims can die of secondary complications a few minutes or up to 96 hours after the incident. Aspiration pneumonia is a late complication of near-drowning episodes, occurring after 48 to 72 hours have elapsed.

Ice Rescue

Attempt to reach the person from shore with a long object (e.g., a branch, a rope, or a board). If there is no equipment, form a human chain reaching from the shore. Lie flat to distribute the weight. Seek medical attention immediately for someone who has fallen through broken ice.

Confined Spaces

A confined space is any area not intended for human occupancy and that also has the potential for containing or accumulating a dangerous atmosphere. Examples of a confined space include a tank, vessel, vat, silo, bin, vault, trench, or pit.

An accident in a confined space demands immediate action. Here is how you can save an entrant's life if that person signals for help or becomes unconscious:

- Call for immediate help.
- Do *not* rush in to help.
- If you are the attendant, do *not* enter the confined space unless:
    1. You are relieved by another attendant, *and*
    2. You are part of the rescue team.
- When help arrives, try to rescue the victim without entering the space.

- If rescue from the outside cannot be done, the trained and properly equipped (respiratory protection plus a safety harness or lifeline) rescuers must enter the space and remove the victim.
- Activate the local emergency medical service (EMS).
- Administer first aid, rescue breathing, or CPR if necessary and if you are trained.

Appendix A
Medicine Chest and First Aid Supplies

Medicine Chest

It is a good idea to have useful medical supplies on hand for emergencies and to treat minor ills, but the family medicine chest does not have to be a mini-drugstore. What should be kept in the average household depends on the makeup of the family.

Generally, medicine chests should include only those health care products likely to be used on a regular basis. A person rarely bothered by constipation, for instance, would have little need for a laxative.

Some drug products lose their potency on the shelf in time, especially after they are opened. Other drugs change in consistency. Milk of magnesia, for instance, dries out if it remains on the shelf for a while after opening. Buying the large "family size" of a product infrequently used may seem like a bargain, but it is poor economy if it has to be thrown out before the contents are used up. Ideally, supplies in the medicine chest should be bought to last over a period of no more than twelve months.

Obviously, selecting health care items for the family medicine chest is a matter of common sense. Here are some suggested items that will meet the needs of most families:

Nondrug Products

Adhesive bandages of assorted sizes
Sterile gauze in pads and a roll
Absorbent cotton
Adhesive tape
Elastic bandage
Small blunt-end scissors
Tweezers
Fever Thermometer, including rectal type for young child
Hot water bottle
Heating pad
Ice bag
Dosage spoon (common household teaspoons are rarely the correct dosage size)
Vaporizer or humidifier

Drug Items

Analgesic (aspirin and/or acetaminophen. Both reduce fever and relieve pain, but only aspirin can reduce inflammation.)
Emetic (syrup of ipecac to induce vomiting and activated charcoal. Read the instructions on how to use these products.)
Antacid
Antiseptic solution
Hydrocortisone creams for skin problems
Calamine for poison ivy and other skin irritations
Petroleum jelly as a lubricant
Antidiarrheic
Cough syrup (nonsuppressant type)
Decongestant
Antibacterial topical ointment
Seasonal items (e.g., insect repellents and sunscreens)

When it comes to storing these health care items, the cardinal rule is to keep all medicines out of the reach of children. In addition, be sure all medications have child-resistant caps. Elderly people who have difficulty opening such caps can ask the pharmacist for caps with regular closure. However, they should be extra careful to see that young visitors cannot get to these drugs.

Both prescription and nonprescription drugs should be kept in a cool, dry place away from foods and other household products. Some drugs may require refrigeration. This should be indicated on the label. If in doubt, ask the pharmacist.

Many people keep medicines on a high shelf in a hall or bedroom closet. Some experts suggest using a locking box. A tackle box might do. A word of warning, however: Be sure all responsible adults in the family know where the key is kept.

To avoid confusion keep prescription and nonprescription drugs in separate boxes clearly labeled to distinguish one type of drug from another. A list of what is in each box, attached to the outside if possible, will make it easier to find specific items, particularly in an emergency.

The medicine chest should be checked periodically to be sure supplies are adequate and to get rid of drugs that may have gone bad or become outdated. Many drug labels have an expiration date beyond which the product should not be used. If there is no date, put a label on the container with the date of purchase and the date it was first opened. Then, if there are any questions in the future, a pharmacist can tell whether the product is safe to use.

Tablets that have become crumbly and medicines that have changed color, odor, or consistency, or are outdated should be destroyed. Empty the bottle of medicine into the toilet, flush it down, and rinse out the bottle. Do not put leftover drugs in the trash basket, where they can be dug out by inquisitive youngsters. Newly purchased drug products that do not look right should be returned to the pharmacy. Drug products that have lost their labels should also be destroyed.

Keep the telephone numbers of the local poison control center, physician, hospital, rescue squad, and fire and police departments near every phone in the house. Tape the emergency phone list inside the bathroom medicine cabinet door, and also keep it with the emergency supplies.

Each family's medicine chest is bound to contain some different items. For help in selecting appropriate health care products, check with a physician and a pharmacist.

Suggested First Aid Kit Contents

Activated charcoal
Adhesive strip bandages, assorted sizes
Adhesive tape, 1- and 2-inch rolls
Alcohol, rubbing (70%)
Alcohol wipes
Antacid
Antibiotic skin ointment (mycin family or triple antibiotic)
Baking soda
Calamine lotion
Chemical ice pack
Cotton balls
Cotton swabs
Decongestant tablets and spray
Diarrhea medication
Disposable gloves, latex
Elastic bandages, 2-, 3-, and 4-inch widths
Extractor™ (Sawyer Products)
Face mask with one-way valve
National Safety Council's First Aid Guide
Flashlight (small) and extra batteries
Gauze pads, 2 × 2 and 4 × 4 inches
Glutose™ (concentrated sugar)
Hot-water bottle
Household ammonia
Hydrocortisone cream (1%)
Hydrogen peroxide
Hypoallergenic tape
Ice bag (plastic)
Insect repellant
Matches

Measuring cup and spoons
Moleskin
Needles
Non-adhering dressing
Oil of cloves
Over-the-counter pain medication (aspirin and acetaminophen)
Over-the-counter antihistamine
Paper and pencil
Paper drinking cups
Roller, self-adhering gauze, 3- and 4-inch widths
Rubber tubing
Safety pins, various sizes
Salt
Scissors
Soap
Space blanket
Spenco 2nd Skin™
SAM Splint™
Sugar
Sunscreen
Syrup of ipecac
Thermometer—1 oral, 1 rectal
Tongue blades
Triangular bandages, 3 or 4
Tweezers
Waterproof tape
Zinc oxide

These items can be placed in a fishing tackle box for storage and transporting.

Appendix B

References to OSHA First Aid Guidelines

Eight OSHA standards have first aid requirements. These guidelines provide institutions teaching first aid courses, and consumers of these courses, what OSHA considers basic and essential elements of a first aid program. These guidelines can also assist compliance officers evaluating individual plant first aid programs during the inspection process.

OSHA does not teach first aid courses, or certify first aid training courses for instructors or trainees.

OSHA standards including first aid provisions:

- General Industry (CFR 1910.151)
- Construction (CFR 1926.50)
- Shipyard (CFR 1915.98)
- Longshoring (CFR 1918.96)
- Diving (CFR 10910.410)
- Hazardous Waste and Emergency Response (CFR 1910.120)
- Temporary Labor Camps (CFR 1910.142)
- First Aid and Lifesaving Facilities (CFR 1914.26)

Appendix C

Resuscitation Masks/ Mouth-to-Barrier Devices

Rescuers should not fear getting a disease, but many may be unwilling to help a person in need because of this fear. For their protection, rescuers should learn resuscitation masks/mouth-to-barrier device use.

Two types of resuscitation masks (mouth-to-barrier devices) exist: mask devices and face shields.

1. Mask devices. Mask devices varying in size, shape, and features are available. For example, some masks allow the delivery of supplemental oxygen. All have a one-way valve so that exhaled air does not enter the rescuer's mouth. The rescuer does not have direct contact with the victim's mouth.

Use the mask by:
a. Attaching the mouthpiece to the mask.
b. Placing the mask on the victim's face so that the top is over the bridge of the nose and the base is between the lower lip and chin.
c. Bend the head back to open the airway. If you suspect a spinal cord injury, follow the procedures in chapter 3.
d. Using both hands to hold the mask firmly in place while keeping the head properly tilted. Do this by placing both thumbs on the sides of the mask and the other fingers grasping the lower jaw. Keep a tight seal around the mask.
e. Placing your mouth over the mouthpiece and blowing into the victim through the mouthpiece.
f. After each breath into the mouthpiece, removing your mouth from it and allowing exhalation from the victim.

Use on infants by reversing the mask so its nose part is under the chin.

The mask can be cleaned in warm soapy water and rinsed in clean water. Then, submerge for 10 minutes in a 1:64 household bleach:water solution before reusing. The one-way valve and filter must be disposed of after using on a victim. Refer to the mask's cleaning instructions for details.

2. Face shields. These are thin, clear plastic devices placed over the mouth of the victim. They prevent contact between the mouths of the rescuer and victim. The mask's clear plastic enables the rescuer to observe vomit.

Use the shield by:
a. Inserting the breathing tube into the victim's mouth until the barrier is touching the victim's lips and face.
b. Bend the head back to open the airway (head-tilt/chin-lift). If you suspect a spinal cord injury, follow the procedures in chapter 3.
c. Placing your fingers under the shield and pinching the victim's nose shut.

The shields are for single use only, do not reuse.

Appendix D
Two Rescuer CPR Procedures

Entry of Second Trained Rescuer to Perform Two-Rescuer CPR	#1 Performing one-rescuer CPR
	
	#2 Says:
	• "I know CPR"
	• "EMS has been activated"
	• "Can I help?"
	
	#1 • Completes CPR cycle (15 compressions and ends on 2 breaths)
	• Says "take over compressions"
	• Checks pulse and breathing (5 seconds)
	• If pulse absent, #1 rescuer says "no pulse, continue CPR"
	
	#2 • Gives 5 compressions (at 80–100 per minute rate)
	• After every 5th compression, pauses for #1 rescuer to give 1 full breath
	
	#1 • Monitors victim while #2 performs compressions:
	    (a) watches chest rise during breaths
	    (b) feels carotid pulse during compressions
	• Gives 1 full breath after every 5th compression given by #2 rescuer

Two Rescuers Starting CPR at the Same Time	#1 (ventilator) • Assesses victim, if no breaths, gives 2 full breaths; if no pulse, tells #2 to start • Gives 1 full breath after every 5th compression by #2 compressions #2 (compressor) • Finds hand position and gets ready to give compressions • Gives 5 compressions after #1 says to start them • Pauses after every 5th compression for #1 to give 1 full breath
Switching During Two-Rescuer CPR	#2 (compressor) • Signals when to change by saying "change and, two and, three and, four and, five" or "change on the next breath" • After #1 gives breath, #2 moves to victim's head and completes pulse and breathing check (5 seconds) and if absent says "no pulse, begin CPR." • Gives a full breath after every cycle of 5 compressions #1 (ventilator) • Gives 1 full breath at the end of 5th compression and moves to victim's chest • Finds hand position and gets ready to give compressions • Begins cycles of 5 compressions after every breath
How an Untrained Rescuer Can Help	• Go for help • Monitor pulse and breathing, with some direction • Give CPR with directions (untrained rescuer can learn compressions easier with trained rescuer giving breaths)

NOTES

Quick Emergency Index